Aromatherapy
& Subtle Energy Techniques

Aromatherapy

& Subtle Energy Techniques

Compassionate Healing with Essential Oils

Joni Keim Loughran & Ruah Bull

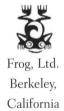

Frog, Ltd.
Berkeley,
California

Aromatherapy & Subtle Energy Techniques
Compassionate Healing with Essential Oils

Published by Frog, Ltd.
Frog, Ltd. Books are distributed by
North Atlantic Books
P. O. Box 12327
Berkeley, California 94712

Book cover and interior designed by Carolina de Bartolo.
Illustrations by Joni Keim Loughran, Carson Chase and Eva Guggemos.
Photos by M. C. Newman

Library of Congress Cataloging-in-Publication Data
 Loughran, Joni.
 Aromatherapy and subtle energy techniques: compassionate healing with essential oils / by Joni Keim Loughran and Ruah Bull.
 p. cm.
 Includes bibliographical references and index.
 ISBN 1-58394-015-4 (alk. paper)
 1. Aromatherapy. 2. Essences and essential oils. 3. Force and energy.
 I. Bull, Ruah, 1951-II. Title.

 RZ999 .L68 2000
 615'.321--dc21   00-026271
                                                              CIP

  1 2 3 4 5 6 7 8 9 / 03 02 01 00

Dedication

Joni Keim Loughran:

To the remarkable women who have meant so much to me:

My mother, Anne Thomas, for her sense of humor and superb ability to make a home.

My sister, Gini, for treasuring our relationship.

My dear friend, Laura, for keeping me young.

My dear friend, Maryann, for her unfailing strength and support.

My soul mate, Patty, who died much too young and told me to go on.

Ruah Bull:

To my husband, Les, dearest friend and companion.

To all my clients, who have taught me what I know about presence, listening, and compassion.

Contents

Contents

Contents

The subtle aromatherapy and energy sessions in this book are intended to assist you and others in promoting a sense of well-being by bringing energetic balance to body and mind. In no way are they intended to supplant professional medical or psychological care.

Acknowledgments

Joni Keim Loughran:
A special thanks to: Gail Atkins for her invaluable help, and for taking the time to edit from a newcomer's point of view. Scott Egide for his encouragement and support. Malte Hozzel for his contributions, vast knowledge, and wisdom. My many aromatherapy instructors and colleagues with whom I've shared the allure and delight of the aromatic path. My teachers in energy healing including Margo Bearheart and Phyllis Schubert. Ruah Bull with whom it has been a great joy and pleasure to create this, our first book.

Ruah Bull:
I want to thank and acknowledge the wonderful staff and faculty at Twin Lakes College of the Healing Arts for the many years of steady friendship and community supporting me as I grew and changed. Special thanks goes to Becky Williams, chosen sister and spiritual friend, for so many things, including my first energy healing class. Thanks to Amber Sharman, aromatherapist and goddess of the office, for insisting I take an aromatherapy class. Thanks to Deb van Dusen and Margo Bearheart for the many conversations about healers and healing. Thanks to all of my students and clients, who taught me how to do this work. Thanks to Joni Keim Loughran, for being my ideal writing partner. And to Spirit—thank you, thank you, thank you.

Foreword

Joni Keim Loughran and Ruah Bull evoke two powerful healing methods, aromatherapy and compassionate touch, and combine them with chakra therapy, auric cleansing, visualization, meditation, and other precious natural approaches to self-healing and self-development. This is more than timely because the physical properties of essential oils have been studied at length during the past two decades, but there has been a lack of the systematic understanding of their subtler workings, and how they might be applied in the field of energy medicine. Joni and Ruah, who are true experts in this area, have done it, and created a book with substantial knowledge for aromatherapy and subtle energy practitioners who want to dig deeper into the finer levels of healing, prevention, and self care.

A work of this kind corresponds to the shift in modern awareness from the matter- and symptom-orientated understanding of medicine which uses synthetic drugs, to the psycho-somatic understanding which takes into account mind-body unity and favors natural and plant-derived medicine. Energy medicine, vibrational healing, subtle body therapies, chakra methods, and aromatherapy are now the next steps, taking us toward a "mind-over-matter" understanding which experiences consciousness as being responsible for our psycho-physiological destiny.

This implies nothing less than the recognition that we are more than mere physical bodies, and that we have to re-introduce the "soul" into both modern science and medicine. It also implies that we acknowledge the existence of the indestructible energy fields around our bodies which reflect our thoughts, emotions, and memories. More than that, we are responsible for these fields and their ability to contribute to the happiness or the suffering of people and the environment around us—healing or polluting, uplifting or degrading. Even science understands now that we communicate more through vibrational or energy exchange than by verbal or body language.

We have to protect this energy field and, if it is disturbed, we can balance and enhance it through energy medicine. In doing this, we can prevent the disturbance from somatizing and becoming dis-ease. This approach is a quantum leap for the western mind, but a catching up with truth that is long since overdue. Eastern thought, such as Ayurveda in India or Traditional Chinese Medicine in China, has tried since time immemorial to encompass the cosmic totality of the patient in healing approaches, and emphasized the priority of the "subtle" energies of consciousness over material, the latter being nothing but a form of contraction or condensation of the subtler, finer levels of life.

Charaka, the famous Ayurvedic physician who lived a few thousand years ago, believed that the errors of our intellect or understanding were the primary causes for disease. In this, we realize that we are truly our own preservers as much as we are our own destroyers. Health and disease become a function of our own volition—emotional, cognitive, and memory-related intelligence. As we metabolize our emotions and desires, as we remember, forget, and forgive, and as we increase the scope of our understanding of life processes, relationships, and our evolutionary path, so shall we enjoy long life and happiness.

Chinese medicine states that if people would massage each other more, there would be fewer wars. Montagu or Liedloff have written about those who, due to the lack of loving touch in early childhood, become neurotic, schizoid personalities, exhibiting in their fearful, aggressive substructure a thirst for touch-experience that has never been quenched. In the last century, the mortality of small children in orphanages was extremely high. This was not due to a lack of hygiene, but due to the fact that the little souls were not hatched, not cradled, not touched, and in essence, not loved enough.

We are on the verge of a collective shift in understanding our need for pure, healing touch. Aggression and unnatural behavior have increased to such an extent in modern life that it seems impossible for the individual to survive unharmed. Our culture calls for a return to true nature, to silence, to spirituality, to our God-given right of bliss. Many of the culture pioneers of our time, who carry the messages of new understanding and behavior into the world, are celebrating in an ever increasing exhilaration, the magic of one of the closest encounters human beings can enjoy together on a physical level: the mystical union of the aromatic touch.

The rediscovery of our sense of smell (olfaction) through aromatherapy, and the accompanying changes in our appreciation of natural versus synthetic scents, goes hand in hand with a rediscovery of our sense of touch. In an aromatic touch experience the frontal and posterial doors of the central nervous system are opened simultaneously through smell and touch, activating an incredible symphony of neuronal connections in the brain, brain stem, and spinal cord. This gives rise to a powerful release of neurotransmitters that dissolve our life traumas into the ocean of preconscious bliss, and we know that paradise is lost no more.

Years ago, as a student, I remember discussing whether world cultures could be understood as happier than others in an objective way, and came to the conclusion that happiness was a subjective term, and that in the end, one was not happier than another. Since then, I have changed my thinking and I must say that medicinal plants and essential oils have played a major role in helping me to understand and experience more of the secret realm of bliss in the human soul. William Blake says, "Energy is joy." This is a profound truth, especially if we look at the hidden energies of our mind and body as we experience them in deep meditation, prayer, union with nature, or in compassionate touch with the grace of the essential oils from medicinal plants, our helpers and companions since antiquity.

Plants have always provided for human and animal life. They have nourished with food, given shelter, and furnished clothing. They have supplied us with medicine—time-tested medicine—from the wisdom of the earth combined with the wisdom of the universe. Looking at plants means to look back at millions of years. It fills us with awe if we realize how much time nature has invested to present us with a lavender, a rosemary, a thyme, or a juniper. In their passive, loving way, plants exhibit a grace and beauty which we as human beings often lack. They are truly messengers from beyond, and we owe them our gratitude and love in exchange and, nowadays, ecological ethics.

When nature started the theme of essential oils in the conifer trees two hundred million years ago, the human species was not yet present. Aromatic substances were used by the trees to defend themselves against the increasing numbers of germs, and for territorial identification. But in a spiritual sense we can understand the first aromatic molecules of the conifer family as a promise for future celebrations between plants and man. From here, aromatic light began its quantum dance through the endless chain of ever new and more complex plants and aromatic substances until a full palette of colors was reached, and the rainbows of vegetal and human lives could touch and nourish each other.

Rig Veda, the oldest text of mankind, speaks about plants as having been sent from heaven into material existence for the divine purpose of life and assistance. Plants "feed" in a most harmonious way upon the heavenly vibrations and radiate these into the world. Their essential oils used in aromatherapy are concentrated energy carriers and messengers that nourish all life from an unseen reservoir of light, full forever. Human love is the best expression of this light on earth. There is no better way for essential oils to unfold their full therapeutic energies than by means of an aroma/touch experience received in a pure, spiritual setting, under the warm, loving strokes of the heart.

Essential oils and compassion, communicated through subtle energy therapy, link back to the inner light of universal love, bridging the gulf between matter and energy, helping to join the banks of separation for moments of unity and bliss.

Malte Hozzel
Naturalist and Procurer of Essential Oils
Provence, France
October 1999

Introduction

Those of us concerned about health and well-being can be grateful to be living in this unique time when ancient and traditional forms of healing, from all over the world, are being re-discovered and re-claimed to accompany the incredible technological breakthroughs of modern medicine. By integrating ancestral wisdom and knowledge into our health care choices, we are recognizing and rejuvenating the multi-dimensional nature of human beings—body, mind, and spirit.

This book has combined, in practice, two such forms of healing: aromatherapy and subtle energy therapy. Though each effectively stands alone, they are extraordinary when used together. Each has a rich history, having been used for thousands of years in a variety of cultures for religious, ceremonial, and medicinal purposes. Aromatherapy, the use of aromatics and essential oils, was employed by the early Egyptians, Greeks, and Romans, and is mentioned several times in the Bible. Subtle energy therapy, also known as energy healing, hands-on-healing, or laying-on-of-hands, was practiced centuries ago by the Essenes, and used in ancient times as well as the present day by the Chinese and native Americans. Today, these two remarkable modalities offer us a way to help ourselves and each other.

Throughout the following pages, we use the term healing in its true sense. The verb "to heal" is from the Anglo-Saxon word haelan which means "to make whole." If health is a state of wholeness, then healing is that which promotes, supports, and sustains it. Life's experiences can throw us out of balance, leaving us feeling broken. Yet everyone has the potential to recover, change, and transcend into wholeness. This book teaches how to use aromatherapy and subtle energy techniques together to serve this purpose of restoring well-being and equilibrium. (In the text, we use the terms "giver" and "receiver" as they are an apt description of the interaction during a subtle energy session.)

A good friend recently said, "Life is a team sport." Indeed, life's ups would be less joyous and downs would be more difficult without the support and companionship of our family and friends. We share our lives with many people and in that sharing, we can be of service during times of physical, emotional, mental, or spiritual difficulties by offering to nurture and heal. It is an innate ability—everyone can comfort as well as send healing energy through their hands.

The methods taught in this book are simple, safe, and effective and can be used by anyone of any age. The techniques have been gathered from many years of study and experience to provide a solid foundation for all who want to assist others in this way. As you begin using them, know that you are both pioneering and traditional—a pioneer because you are entering an amazing new arena of help and self-help, and a traditionalist because you are employing age-old traditions and natural skills.

We are all sharing in this extraordinary adventure of re-discovering our natural capacity to heal and be healed. We encourage those of you who want to explore beyond the introductory level of this book and include lists of resources on aromatherapy and subtle energy therapy.

Whether you are a lay person who wants to be of service to friends, family, or community, or a professional who wants to integrate this work into your practice, remember to come to this experience with the playful wonderment, openness, and innocence of a child. We hope that the information and experience we have provided brings you, as it has brought us, great joy.

ONE

Introduction to Subtle Energy Therapy

*T*here is a burgeoning field of therapeutic work being practiced by professionals and lay persons alike known as subtle energy therapy. This is a general term for a variety of methods being used today. Though their philosophies, style, and techniques vary, they are all based on the same principle: that our bodies are electromagnetic and energetic in nature, and this energy can be influenced in a positive/therapeutic way to promote health, balance, and well-being.

The most well-known subtle energy therapies that employ the use of a practitioner's hands are Therapeutic Touch, Reiki, aspects of Polarity, Subtle Energy Medicine, and the teachings of two highly recognized instructors, Earth Energy Healing with Rosalyn Bruyere and Hands-on-Healing with Barbara Brennan. A leading practitioner in each method offers a brief description:

Therapeutic Touch was developed by Dolores Krieger and Dora Kunz in 1972. "To promote healing, the practitioner centers and aligns him/herself to use universal energy as the means to consciously direct or adjust the receiver's energy. It is done by passing the hands over the receiver's body to ascertain any abnormalities, cleansing the energy field, and then directing and balancing the energy."—Calvin Davis

Reiki (ray-key) was founded in the early 1900s by Mikao Usui in Japan, and was brought to the western world by Mrs. Hawayo Takata in the 1940s. "Its name means universal life energy, and it has been used for thousands of years. Reiki was rediscovered by Usui in the 2500-year-old writings of the Tibetan Sutras, and is used today to promote physical, mental, emotional, and spiritual wellness. Practitioners describe its effects as amplifying the innate ability to heal with touch."—Skip James

Polarity Therapy was developed by Dr. Randolph Stone, D.O., D.C., N.D. in the early 1900s. "Dr. Stone studied a variety of modalities, including Ayurveda, yoga, and traditional Western medicine, and integrated them into a new, wholistic health system. Polarity includes body work, nutrition, exercises, and developing a positive attitude."—Jan Fitzgerald

Subtle Energy Medicine is an example of an integrative approach to subtle energy therapy. It is "a method in which the practitioner channels different energy frequencies through their subtle energy body into the receiver's subtle energy system. The receiver takes this energy transmission to revitalize and encourage healing. This system uses an ultrasound frequency that helps the blocked energy of the receiver to open up and receive."—Margo Bearheart

Earth Energy Healing, developed by Rosalyn Bruyere, "is a technique that draws vibrational energy up from the earth that is then channeled through the practitioner's body and hands to impact the physical and etheric body of the receiver. It uses sound as well as light frequencies to bring the system into balance." —Ruah Bull

Hands-on-Healing, developed by Barbara Brennan, uses "the body's innate wisdom and natural instinct to move towards health. A healer trained in this method works with the different dimensions of being: physical, auric, hara, and core star. By using a laying-on-of-hands, the healer releases blocks, balances, and charges the energetic field surrounding the body. This enables one to realign with the creative force which is available to each and everyone."—Betsy Ginkel

The Therapeutic Nature of Compassionate Touch

"The skin of the human being is an extraordinary liminal boundary where inner and outer realities of body and soul meet. In therapeutic body work there is an exceptional opportunity not only to alleviate physical pain and stress, but also to address the deep feeling and suffering of the soul."

—Patricia Kaminski, *Touching the Soul*

Using the hands to touch with the desire to help, promote health, and heal is not new. It is a natural and inherent part of being human, and has been used throughout history. What is more instinctual than to put your hand on an aching knee? Or to hold someone who has been hurt? Or for a mother to cradle her crying baby? Archeologists discovered in the Dead Sea Scrolls that the Essenes trained people in their community to heal with their hands. Native American healers included touch in their ceremonies, and Traditional Chinese Medicine (TCM), in ancient times as well as today, has employed the fundamental principle that hands have the ability to heal.

Using hands in this restorative, benevolent way is a universal language of emotional nourishment that answers a basic, human need. We need to be touched. It is the first of the five senses to develop in human beings, and usually the last to decline. It is an essential part of our well-being, and we thrive from the experience of being connected to another. The May 1999 issue of *Natural Health* reported that premature babies who were massaged were sent home six days earlier than babies who were not; and patients whose hands were held for just thirty seconds before surgery recovered faster than those whose hands were not held. Researchers at the Touch Research Institute at the University of Miami School of Medicine say that a daily dose of touch can be as essential to good health as diet and exercise. Ashley Montague, author of the 1971 ground-breaking book, *Touching: The Human Significance of Skin,* said, "The communication we transmit through touch constitutes the most powerful means

5

of establishing human relationships, the foundation of experience. Where touching begins, there love and humanity also begin . . .." Deborah Cowens, author of *A Gift For Healing,* says it "is the most human of all forms of healing, using the hands to reach out in service to another person in a gesture of peace, balance, and love." She reports that, "Studies have shown that those people receiving healing touch have increased alpha brain waves, characteristic of people in a meditative state. Such deep states of relaxation are associated with diminution of stress, improved respiration, better hormonal balance, lower blood cholesterol levels, and heightened immune response."

Many of the subtle energy techniques described in this book are performed with the giver's hands, using them on or around the receiver, and transmitting healing energy. Combining compassion with an understanding of the body's energetic anatomy complements the hand's ability to give and heal.

Energy Anatomy

Subtle energy is produced by our body's energy anatomy, also referred to as our subtle anatomy. It consists of energy centers and subtle bodies. The seven primary energy centers are located along the spine from the tailbone to the top of the head. These spinning energy centers are often called chakras, a Sanskrit word meaning "wheels of light." They receive, assimilate, and transmit various forms of energy, and play a vital role in our state of consciousness and emotional nature. The energy centers correspond to major aspects of our lives: survival, sex, power, love, communication, intuition, and spirituality. In the *Sevenfold Journey,* Anodea Judith and Selene Vega write, "None of the chakras function by themselves. As wheels spinning at the core of our being, the chakras are intermeshing gears, working together to run the delicate machinery of our lives."

The subtle bodies are levels of energy that permeate through the physical body and continue outward from the skin forming an energetic structure which is perceived as an aura. The aura can extend from a foot to many feet away from the body, the average being about three feet. It is generally described as having four or seven subtle bodies, depending on the source of information. (For our purposes, we will use the four-subtle-body model.) The levels closest to the body are the most dense and have the lowest frequencies. As the levels move away from the body, they become less dense and have higher frequencies. The aura expands with positive thoughts and feelings such as joy and happiness, and contracts with negative feelings such as fear or hatred. The subtle bodies shift constantly in response to life experiences and moods, changing in shape, size, and color.

The Primary Energy Centers

Ideally, the seven primary energy centers spin harmoniously together, clockwise. (The orientation for this clockwise motion is from the outside, looking at the body.) Anodea Judith states in *Eastern Body, Western Mind*, "All of the chakras need to be open, and functioning in balance with the others to be a fully thriving human being." The shape of the spin should be circular, full, and of equal size and consistent shape. The first center, at the base of the spine, points down toward the earth. The seventh center, at the top of the head, opens to the heavens. The others, second through sixth, radiate out from both the front and back of the body, in specific locations. The first, second, and third energy centers located in the lower part of the body represent the physical realm and are related to the elements of earth, water, and fire. The fifth, sixth, and seventh in the upper part represent the spiritual realm. These triads are joined together and balanced by the fourth center, the Heart center, in the middle of the body.

Lesser, or secondary, energy centers are located throughout the body. There is an energy center at every joint such as the knee and hip. Two of the most important secondary chakras are on the hands, which are concerned with creativity when we make or do something, and on the feet, which are concerned with maintaining a connection with the earth and receiving its energy.

At any given time, an energy center can be blocked or thrown out of balance. Fear is a common reason for this to occur, as well as sudden shock, or repressed emotions or feelings. An imbalance in one energy center can affect the others, especially those closest to it. For example, if you experience sudden grief (fourth energy center), it can give you an upset stomach (third energy center) and make it difficult for you to speak (fifth energy center).

Under stressful circumstances—physical, mental, emotional, or spiritual—the energy centers react and reflect the predicament, distorting from their balanced states. The spin can speed up, slow down, or change directions (counter-clockwise); the shape can become contorted; and the size can become smaller (constricted energy) or larger (congested energy).

8

All of these distortions can cause or represent problems that correlate to the various energy centers. For example, a distortion in the fifth center (Throat) could stem from issues related to communication, and may result in physical symptoms such as a sore throat, or psychological symptoms such as difficulty in communicating.

Imbalances or blockages can be eased or corrected by contact with an energy that nurtures, or one that vibrates at that affected center's healthiest frequency. Using subtle energy therapy techniques combined with appropriate essential oils (aromatherapy) serves this purpose well and effectively, facilitating positive change.

The following charts are a general explanation of the seven primary energy centers. At the top of the chart is the common name or names of each center and an affirmation that describes its essence. Following that is the location of the center as it relates to the physical body, and the concerns of each center, thought of as the duties to which they attend. The key concept is italicized. If the center is in balance, it reflects the healthy characteristics specified in "positive state." Imbalanced conditions are also noted, providing clues to understanding which centers might be out of balance and requiring attention. Each center provides energy for and is associated with a gland of the endocrine system, as well as parts of the body. If a center is greatly out of balance, symptoms might be experienced in the associated area. Each energy center responds and relates to a specific color, as listed, benefiting from the color's characteristics. (In Chapter 4 you will learn more about color and how it can be used with subtle energy techniques.)

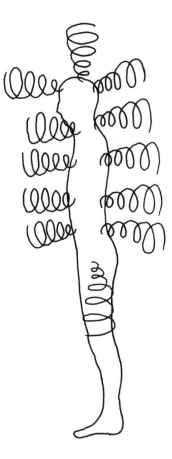

9

First/Root or Base "I am."

Location	Base of spine.
Concerns	Self preservation. Connection to Mother Earth, physical existence, survival, health, security, home, food.
Positive state	Strong relationship with Mother Earth, positive attitude about life, good health, vitality, feeling stable, safe, and secure.
Imbalanced state	Disconnected from body, fearful, disorganized, possessive.
Gland association	Adrenal
Parts of body influenced	Urogenital system, intestines, bones, legs, feet, base of spine.
Color	Clear red (revitalizing)

Second/Sacral "I want. I create. I desire."

Location	Two inches below the navel.
Concerns	Self gratification. Sexuality, creativity, desire, reproduction, personal growth, pleasure, emotions, relationships.
Positive state	Comfortable flow of feelings, enthusiasm about life, creative actions, capable of feeling sexual and sensual pleasure.
Imbalanced state	Sexual problems, mood swings, emotionally dependent or detached, lack of self-love.
Gland association	Reproductive (Ovaries for females, testes for males)
Parts of body influenced	Urogenital system, reproductive organs, urinary system, lower back.
Color	Clear orange (energizing)

Third/Solar Plexus "I manifest."

Location	Two inches above the navel.
Concerns	Personal identity. Personality, personal power and will, energy, self-worth, likes and dislikes, social identity, beliefs, attitudes, activities.
Positive state	Inner harmony, self-acceptance, confidence, comfortable with life experiences, attracting what you want in life, warm personality, responsible.
Imbalanced state	Low self-esteem, temper outbursts, stubbornness, hyperactivity, trying too hard to please, unable to express anger.
Gland association	Pancreas
Parts of body	Digestive system, stomach, pancreas, gall bladder, liver, middle back.
Color	Clear yellow (invigorating)

Fourth/Heart "I love."

Location	Center of chest.
Concerns	Acceptance of self and others. Love, empathy, sympathy, compassion, connects lower and upper energy centers, appreciation of the arts, one's life purpose, connection with friends and family, good will, devotion.
Positive state	Radiates warmth and sincerity, ability to nurture oneself and others, gives with joy, altruistic, peaceful.
Imbalanced state	Love and intimacy problems, anti-social tendencies, depression, jealousy.
Gland association	Thymus
Parts of body influenced	Circulatory system, heart, lungs, arms, breasts, upper back.
Color	Clear green (regenerating), and pink (loving)

Fifth/Throat "I speak my truth."

Location	Center of throat.
Concerns	Self expression. Communication (listening & speaking), creativity, alignment of personal will with Divine will, time management.
Positive state	Freely expresses feelings, good listener, speaks clearly, involved in creative activities.
Imbalanced state	Shyness, fear of speaking, talks too much, inability to listen, rushed—not enough time.
Gland association	Thyroid, parathyroid
Parts of body influenced	Respiratory system, throat, mouth, ears, neck, nose.
Color	Clear sky blue (soothing)

Sixth/Third Eye or Brow "I see. I understand."

Location	Center of forehead.
Concerns	Self reflection. Intellect, perception, mental clarity, dreams, memory, intuition, understanding, imagination.
Positive state	Active intelligence, intuitive, good memory, interested in spirituality, perceptive.
Imbalanced state	Forgetful, impaired vision, overly mental, experiences nightmares.
Gland association	Pituitary, hypothalamus
Parts of body influenced	Central nervous system, head, eyes, brain, face.
Color	Clear indigo blue (opening)

Seventh/Crown *"I am one with the Divine."*

Location	Top of head.
Concerns	Self knowledge. Sense of oneness, complete understanding, spirituality, faith, higher states of consciousness, divinity.
Positive state	Open-minded, balanced with other energy centers, unites inner and outer life, Divinely guided actions, spiritual, thoughtful, wise.
Imbalanced state	Apathetic, fear of death, lack of life purpose, disassociation with body.
Gland association	Pineal
Parts of body influenced	Central nervous system, brain.
Color	Clear violet (transforming), and white (integrating)

The Subtle Bodies

The subtle bodies, also known as the energy field, auric field, or electro-magnetic field, play a vital role in our health, providing energy for the seven primary energy centers that will, in turn, be used by the physical body. Dr. Richard Gerber, author of *Vibrational Medicine,* states, "It is becoming increasingly clear that it is possible to therapeutically impact upon physical and emotional illness by affecting the higher frequency structures [subtle bodies] which are in dynamic equilibrium with the physical body." For our purposes, we use a four-subtle-body system.

The etheric body lies directly outside of the physical body. It has a direct correlation with the state of the physical body and all of its sensations. The etheric body sustains the equilibrium between the physical body and the other subtle bodies, and houses an exact energetic replica of the physical body, providing a blueprint. This level is strengthened by good health, including physical exercise.

14

The astral body houses our feelings and emotions, and our relationships with people, animals, plants, our environment, and the universe. It affects the physical body through the nervous, endocrine, muscular, and immune systems. Positive emotions (love, joy, hope) expand the field while negative emotions (fear, anger, hatred) contract it. This level is strong when feelings, both negative and positive, are allowed to flow (not repressed), and when we have good relationships with people, giving importance to family, friends, and community.

The mental body houses intellectual function, rational thoughts, beliefs, judgements, the conscious and unconscious mind, and memories. This level is strengthened by activities such as learning, studying, and meditating.

The spiritual body houses our spiritual essence, and the knowing of one's life purpose. It connects us to our spiritual self and emotional experiences of Divine love, spiritual joy, and bliss. The spiritual body organizes the subtle bodies and holds them in association with the physical body. It provides a protective boundary where our energy ends and the rest of the world begins. This level is strengthened by maintaining harmony in our lives, seeking higher truths, feeling connected to a greater purpose, and knowing we are a part of a Divine plan.

Rosalyn Bruyere, author of *Wheels of Light,* explains that an abnormality in the auric field can be a warning that something is wrong in the physical body even though there may not yet be physical symptoms. She believes that dis-ease manifests first in the subtle bodies on an energetic level, and then condenses to manifest in the physical body. If a disturbance is detected and treated in the subtle bodies, dis-ease and disharmony in the physical body can be helped or prevented. Existing problems also can be influenced and assisted by working with the subtle bodies. To this end, subtle energy therapy uses the hands with intention, imagination, and creativity to direct healing energy in and around the body to produce a positive change.

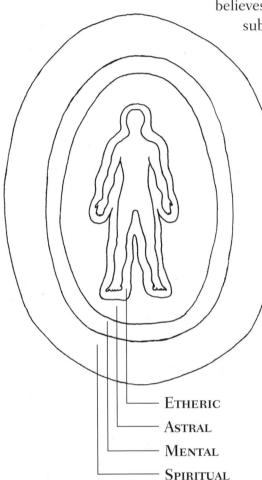

ETHERIC

ASTRAL

MENTAL

SPIRITUAL

15

Exercises

Feeling Energy in Your Hands

Throughout this book, you will read about energy, our nature as energetic human beings, and healing with energy. This exercise is designed to help you feel and experience this energy as it is sensed between your hands.

Sit or stand comfortably and take a few deep breaths.

Hold your hands about 2 feet apart, and slowly bring them together. Notice any sensations as they approach and finally touch each other.

Vigorously rub your hands together to build energy, then move them 3 inches apart, noticing any sensations.

Rub them together vigorously again. Move them 3 inches apart, then 6 inches, then 12 inches, and notice what you feel.

From 6 inches apart, pump your hands together and apart, slowly, several times. Imagine an "energy ball" forming between your hands.

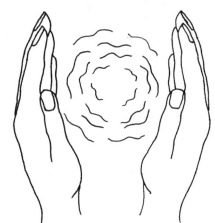

Experiment with moving your hands closer together and farther apart. How do you experience feeling the energy? Some people feel a type of tingling or warmth while others sense a thickness, as if holding a balloon. Remember, one perception is not better than another and there is no right or wrong way of sensing.

Sensing the Auric Field

For this exercise you will need a partner. Because most people cannot see the auric field, this exercise is helpful to practice feeling it.

Have your partner stand or sit comfortably 8-10 feet away from you.

Take a few moments to do the above exercise, "Feeling Energy in Your Hands".

Now, hold your hands out in front of you, palms facing forward, in a comfortable position. Slowly approach your partner. As you get closer to

16

the physical body, notice what you feel or sense. You may notice a change in density or temperature, or sense a slight resistance. This usually happens when you reach the etheric level, which is just a few inches away from the physical body.

Continue moving toward your partner and gently touch them. Ask your partner to close their eyes, and to let you know when they can first feel your presence. This is usually before the actual physical touch.

Begin slowly moving away again. Pay attention to any subtle shifts as you sense the transitions between the different levels of the auric field.

Repeat this approach-and-back-away technique a few more times. Most beginners are able to sense the etheric body fairly easily with practice. Acknowledge your own style of experiencing the energy of the auric field. Some people have a "feeling" sensation, others have a sense of "knowing," and still others experience images or colors.

Energy Center Meditation

This is a lovely exercise to increase your awareness of your energy centers while you nurture and support each one. Find a quiet, private place. You will need about fifteen minutes, without interruption. Sit in a comfortable, relaxed position with your back supported. Your spine should be as straight as possible. Take a few, deep, relaxing breaths, and become aware of your whole body. Then imagine your whole body comfortable and relaxed.

Let your awareness move into your first energy center at the base of your spine. Visualize, feel, or imagine a clear red light facing down into the earth, spinning clockwise,* round and full. Let this red color become vibrant. Repeat a phrase that nourishes this energy center, and is meaningful to you such as, "I am safe," "I am secure," or "I trust the universe." Feel grounded and connected with Mother Earth and enjoy this sensation.

*Use the following technique to determine which direction is clockwise: Put your right thumb in the center of an energy center of your choice, such as the Solar Plexus. The direction your fingers are pointing is the clockwise direction of the spin.

Move your awareness to your second energy center, two inches below your navel. Imagine a clear orange light, spinning clockwise, shining out the front and back of your body. The shape of the center is round and full, and the same size as your first center. Repeat a phrase that nourishes this center, and is meaningful to you. For example, "I feel my emotions," "I am creative," "I know what I want and desire," or "I deserve pleasure." Feel comfortable with and connected to your creative, emotional, and sexual self.

Move your awareness to your third energy center, two inches above your navel. Create a beautiful clear yellow light, spinning clockwise, shining out of the front and back of your body, similar in shape and size to the first two centers. Repeat a meaningful phrase such as, "I manifest what I want to accomplish," or "I am a worthy, competent, beautiful human being." Affirm your personal power and will.

Move your awareness to the fourth energy center, the Heart, in the middle of your chest. Visualize a clear green or pink light shining out the front and back of your body, spinning clockwise. Once again, it is round and full, the same size and shape as the others. Strengthen and affirm this center by repeating a meaningful phrase such as, "I am lovable," "I love others unconditionally," or "I know how to tend to myself and to others." Feel a capacity for compassion and unconditional love.

Move your awareness to the center of your throat at the fifth energy center. Create a clear, sky blue light spinning clockwise, radiating out the front and back of your neck. It is the same size and shape as the others. Repeat a meaningful phrase that affirms your capacity to speak, listen, and live with integrity such as, "I speak my truth," "I listen carefully to others," or "I have enough time to do the things that are important to me." Experience and enjoy being with what is true for you.

Move your awareness to the center of your forehead at the sixth energy center, also known as the Third Eye. Imagine a deep, clear, indigo blue light shining out the front and back of your head, spinning clockwise, and the same shape and size as the others. Repeat a phrase that is meaningful to you that supports this center such as, "I see and understand," "I have an excellent mind that is both intuitive and rational," or "My imagination supports my creativity and perceptiveness." Appreciate and affirm your mental capacities.

Move your awareness to the top of your head at the seventh energy center also known as the Crown. Experience a clear violet or white light, round and full, spinning clockwise, shining up to the heavens. It is the same size and shape as the others. Repeat a supporting and strengthening phrase such as, "I am one with the Divine," "I am walking my soul path," or "I am open to receiving the wisdom of the universe." Enjoy being aware of your deepest and highest spirituality.

Take a few moments to experience all of your energy centers, spinning harmoniously together. Sense how your body radiates the clear colors like a rainbow. Visualize the centers becoming the size appropriate for you to return to your daily activities—not too open and not too closed. Look forward to being balanced, knowing your energy centers are drawing in and distributing all the energy they need. Take a few, deep, re-orienting breaths, open your eyes, and feel relaxed, refreshed, fully in your body, and fully appreciating who you are.

19

Resources

We encourage our readers to seek further education in the field of subtle energy therapy. We believe that learning is a lifelong journey that is both rewarding and enjoyable. The following are resources for the subtle energy therapies mentioned at the beginning of this chapter. We have included a practitioner as well as an association or school, when available, for you to contact.

Therapeutic Touch
Calvin Reed Davis
707-823-6919
Calvin Davis is certified in Therapeutic Touch, Jin Shin Jyutsu, Reflexology, and Aromatherapy.

Nurse Healers-Professional Association Cooperative, Inc.
175 Fifth Avenue, Suite 2755
New York, New York 10010

Reiki
Skip James
831-457-8009
Skip is a certified massage therapist, hypnotherapist, Reiki practitioner, and teacher. He is the developer of Jiva Shanta Reiki.

Universal Reiki Association
128 Fugus St.
Santa Cruz, CA 95062
831-251-0784
universalreikias@aol.com

Polarity Therapy
Jan Fitzgerald
831-429-2204
Jan Fitzgerald is a certified massage therapist, hypnothera-
pist, and aromatherapist. She has a Ph.D. in Educational
Linguistics.

American Polarity Therapy Association
2888 Bluff St. #149
Boulder, CO 80301

Subtle Energy Medicine
Reverend Margo Bearheart
707-579-0737
Email: www.bearhart@sonic.net
Rev. Bearheart is the founder and director of the
Transformational Healing Arts Center. She has been teach-
ing classes and trainings for over twenty-five years.

The Transformational Healing Arts Center
709 Davis Street
Santa Rosa, CA 95401

Earth Energy Healing
Ruah Bull
707-762-3404
Email: ruahb@earthlink.net
Ruah integrates hypnosis, energy healing, aromatherapy,
and spiritual direction in her practice. She has been teaching and in private practice since 1978.

Rosalyn Bruyere's Healing Light Center Church
261 E. Allegria, #12
Sierra Madre, CA 91025

Hands-on-Healing
Betsy Ginkel
707-769-8801
Betsy is an experienced practitioner of the Barbara Brennan
School of Healing.

Barbara Brennan's School of Healing
P.O. Box 2005
East Hampton, NY 11937

Energy Bodywork
(Including Polarity, Reiki, Hands-on-Healing)
Twin Lakes College of the Healing Arts
1210 Brommer St.
Santa Cruz, CA 95062
831-476-2152

Recommended Reading

Eastern Body, Western Mind, Anodea Judith (New York: Harper Row, 1998).

The Sevenfold Journey, Anodea Judith and Selene Vega (Freedom, CA: Crossing Press, 1993).

Anatomy of the Spirit, Carolyn Myss (New York: Harmony Books, 1996).

Wheels of Light, Roselyn Bruyere (New York: Simon and Schuster, 1994).

Hands of Light, Barbara Ann Brennan (New York: Bantam Books, 1988).

Vibrational Medicine, Richard Gerber, M. D. (Santa Fe, NM: Bear & Company, 1988).

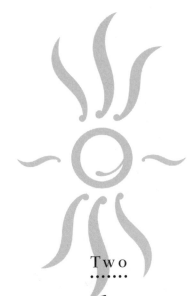

Two

Introduction
to Aromatherapy

$\mathcal{A}$romatherapy is the art and science of using the therapeutic properties of fragrant, concentrated plant extracts known as essential oils to promote health and well-being. Related to herbal therapy, it has been used for thousands of years by many cultures for religious, ceremonial, and medical purposes. Today, essential oils are being used to treat physical, psychological, and energetic (including spiritual) imbalances and have become increasingly popular as interest in self-care and natural products grows. Essential oils are effective only if they are pure and unadulterated, and extracted from plants that have been properly grown, harvested, and distilled. Most essential oils are complex, and their unique, therapeutic properties cannot be synthetically duplicated in a laboratory.

On a physical level, essential oils are used both medically and cosmetically. In a medical context, they can relieve cold and flu symptoms when used in massages, baths, compresses, or inhalations. Essential oils are versatile in their physical and medical applications, and have many properties that can be employed to relieve pain, reduce inflammation, relax muscles, support the immune system, promote wound healing, stimulate circulation, and kill bacteria, fungi, and viruses. In France, the center for medical applications of essential oils, aromatherapy is taught to medical students and is used by both doctors and nurses. Eucalyptus, lavender, and tea tree essential oils are commonly used in medical applications.

Cosmetically, essential oils are used to nurture and rejuvenate the complexion. They are a boon to skin care because their small molecular structure allows them to penetrate into the deeper layers of the dermis where they can be truly effective. All types of skin, from oily to mature, can benefit. Essential oils help to balance glandular activity, promote cellular regeneration, soothe and calm irritations, and stimulate circulation. They are used in facial cleansers, toners, moisturizers, masks, and mists. Lavender, neroli, ylang ylang, chamomile, and geranium are common cosmetic essential oils, imparting beautiful fragrances as well as restorative properties.

In a psychological context, aromatherapy is used to reduce stress and relieve negative mental states such as depression, anxiety, anger, and fear. This can be achieved in two different ways: by choosing an essential oil with the correct properties such as lavender, chamomile, neroli, or clary sage for relaxation and relieving anxiety when used in a bath or massage; and by using memory and association with a scent to re-create positive feelings. In the latter case, a pleasant-smelling essential oil is used in conjunction with a pleasant experience such as smelling jasmine or rose while enjoying a stroll in your garden or having a massage. If repeated, the pleasant experience and the scent will be locked together into your memory. When this happens, you can simply smell the essential oil and it will re-create the positive feelings associated with the pleasant experience. Some people like to use the same massage oil every time they receive a massage. Afterwards, when they smell the oil, they experience a sense of relaxation and nurturing. An association can be created to relieve stress, fear, or other contrary feelings.

On an energetic level, which is the focus of this book, essential oils are used to affect the auric field and the energy centers of the body. Essential oils are well-suited to assist meditations, affirmations, visualizations, and other transformative techniques that benefit from the vibrational or frequency qualities of essential oils.

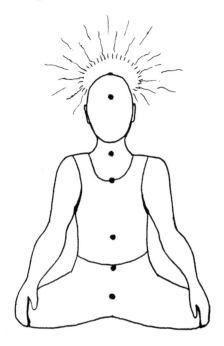

The History of Aromatherapy

R.M. Gattefossé, a French chemist and perfumer, is considered the father of modern day aromatherapy. In the early 1920s, Gattefossé seriously burned his hand in the laboratory, and quickly immersed it in the only liquid available, a vat of lavender oil. To his amazement, the burn lost its redness and the pain diminished rapidly. As days passed, it healed much sooner than expected. He was so impressed with this reaction that he began investigating the medicinal properties of essential oils and dedicated the rest of his life to this research, coining the term "aromatherapy" in 1928.

There was some initial interest in the work of Gattefossé but when World War II erupted, it declined. Real interest began with Dr. Jean Valnet's book, *Aromatherapie: The Treatment of Illness with the Essence of Plants,* published in 1964. A French medical doctor, Valnet was inspired by Gattefossé's research. He used antiseptic essential oils to treat wounds and infections, to fumigate hospital wards, and to sterilize surgical instruments. Two of Valnet's students, Margarite Maury and Micheline Archier, brought aromatherapy to England, using it for massage and skin care. Madame Maury later became respected for her research on both the physical and psychological effects of essential oils.

In 1977, Robert Tisserand discovered Valnet's book on a visit to France from his native England. He translated it, and published *The Art of Aromatherapy* in 1979, bringing the book to the English speaking world. This book is now available in seven languages. In the late 1980s, aromatherapy gained a strong foothold in the United States, led by Kurt Schnaubelt, Marcel Lavabre, and Victoria Edwards. The National Association of Holistic Aromatherapy emerged as a strong fellowship of interested professionals and lay people, advocating aromatherapy as a self-help modality. The 1990s have brought continued interest, commercial growth, and research, substantiating aromatherapy's applications and effectiveness. Germany is known for its scientific and chemical research, France for its medical applications, England for massage and skin care, Italy for psychology, and the United States for its diverse use and quality education.

The Nature of Essential Oils

Essential oils are an extraordinary gift from the plant kingdom. Highly concentrated, they are up to one hundred times stronger than the dried herb of the same plant. They exist in a variety of colors and viscosities. For instance, bergamot is green and watery while benzoin is amber and thick. They will last for many years when properly stored in dark, glass bottles with tight fitting caps, and away from heat and light. Essential oils are not oils in a true sense because they do not contain fatty acids, and for this reason, they do not become rancid. They are volatile, evaporating into the air if left in an open container. This volatility is why they have also been called etheric oils.

The quality and properties of an essential oil depend on the soil in which the plant is grown, as well as the climate, location, amount of sun exposure, amount of water received, time of extraction, and type of distillation. Some plants produce an abundance of essential oils while others produce very little. The concentration of essential oil in the plant, and how it is extracted will ultimately dictate its price. For example, peppermint and citrus produce large amounts of essential oil and are relatively inexpensive. Rose produces very little, taking up to three thousand pounds of petals to produce one pound of oil, and as a result, it is one of the most expensive oils.

Various plant parts produce different essential oils. Flowers are used for rose, leaves for sage, roots for vetiver, fruit seeds for coriander, wood for

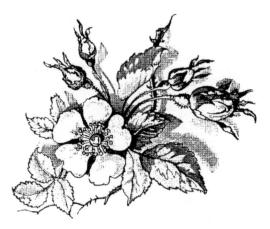

sandalwood, bark for cinnamon, resin for myrrh, and rind for citrus oils such as orange, lemon, and lime. Interestingly, there are a few plants that produce different essential oils from different parts of the same plant. The bitter orange tree produces three different oils: orange oil from the rind of the fruit, petitgrain from the leaves and twigs, and neroli from the blossoms.

Essential oils must be carefully extracted at the right stage of plant development, using the right method of extraction, in order to preserve the oil's valuable therapeutic properties. The method of extraction must suit the plant while protecting the essential oil. The most common is steam distillation. During this method, the fresh plant is placed in a vessel where steam is released into it. The steam and the essential oil rise from the vessel and are condensed. As they flow through a refrigerated coil into another container, they separate into two parts: the oily part known as the essential oil and the watery part known as the hydrosol. Cold expression extraction is used for citrus. In this case, the rind is shredded, sometimes mixed with a little water and then extracted by pressure. Other methods include the use of solvents, and carbon dioxide. Experimentation continues looking for new, more effective methods of extraction to obtain an oil while preserving its natural and complete properties.

31

How Essential Oils Affect Us

Essential oils are used to restore health and well-being via skin (dermal) application and inhalation (odor molecules entering the nose). The most common methods are massages, baths, compresses, and diffusion. Their small molecular structure and attraction-to-oil (lipophilic) characteristics allow them to be absorbed quickly and easily into the skin where they enter the blood stream through small capillaries, circulate throughout the body, and are eliminated through the sweat glands and normal body functions. Most essential oils begin circulating about twenty minutes after application, and can continue for as long as twenty-four hours. Interestingly, however, the memory of the scent and the experience associated with it can last a lifetime.

When the scent of an essential oil is inhaled through the nose, certain odor molecules enter the lungs and others travel to the brain. If through the lungs, the odor molecules enter the blood stream and circulate through the body, as described above. Those traveling to the brain are perceived by our sense of smell and have a profound effect, producing emotional responses, memories, instinctual drives, and even affecting glandular functions via the hypothalamus. Anthropologist Lauren Van Der Post said, "Scent . . . is not only biologically the oldest but also the most evocative of all our senses. It goes deeper than conscious thought or organized memory and has a will of its own which human imagination is compelled to obey."

When a scent enters the nose, it goes through three stages, all happening in a split second:

Reception: Odor molecules bind to the olfactory epithelium inside the top of the nose. The epithelium contains more than ten million nerve endings that respond to specific aromatic molecules.

Transmission: Nerve impulses are sent to the olfactory bulb at the base of the brain which then sends impulses to the cerebral cortex and the limbic system. Nerve messages from our sense of smell travel faster to the brain than those from any of our other senses.

Perception: The message is received by the limbic system which is the seat of emotions and memory, and consists mainly of: the amygdala, which houses instinctual behavior, emotions, memories; the hypothalamus, which controls the autonomic nervous system, body temperature, hunger, and thirst; and the pituitary, which receives messages from the hypothalamus and sends chemical messengers into the blood, releasing hormones that regulate body functions.

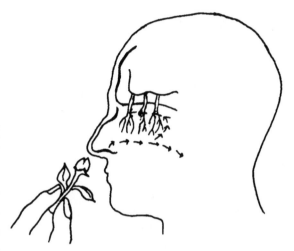

Essential oils are selected for therapeutic purposes based primarily on their chemical make-up. The chemical constituents in an essential oil are largely responsible for its properties and purpose, having unique capabilities and producing effects that can calm, sedate, stimulate, regenerate, reduce inflammation, or inhibit bacteria. For example, oxides have expectorant qualities, making them useful for colds and congestion, and are found in tea tree, rosemary, and eucalyptus oils. Aldehydes reduce inflammation and are calming, and are found in lemongrass, lemon verbena, and melissa. Esters are a valuable group of components that balance and soothe, and are contained in lavender, clary sage, geranium, and Roman chamomile. When essential oils are correctly chosen, the desired results can be realized.

The energetic nature of essential oils make them useful for subtle energy therapy. In this case, energetic imbalances are addressed, and not necessarily physical symptoms. This energetic quality is not based on the chemical constituents of the oil alone. They are based on a variety of information which will be discussed at length in Chapter 3.

33

Methods of Using Essential Oils

Generally, essential oils are used diluted because they are so concentrated, and can be irritating to the skin if used full strength, however, there are exceptions to this. Some oils and particular situations call for using essential oils undiluted (neat). A drop of lavender can be applied to insect bites or small burns; a drop of peppermint on the temples can help relieve a headache; and a drop of tea tree can be applied for fungal infections.

There are a variety of ways to use essential oils: inhalations, baths, massages, compresses, or misters.

Inhalations

Hot water method. Add two to three drops of essential oils to a bowl of very hot water, wait one minute, then cover your head with a towel as you lean over the bowl. Close your eyes and breathe deeply and gently through your nose for two minutes.

Diffusers. Follow the manufacturer's instructions. Diffusers disperse odor molecules into the air by cool air or gentle warmth. Use for ten to fifteen minutes per hour. Thick oils such as sandalwood, benzoin, and vetiver cannot be used in some diffusers unless first mixed with lighter oils. Use only pure essential oils. Do not dilute in a carrier oil because it will not diffuse properly and can clog some diffusers.

Direct. Smell out of the bottle, or from a tissue dabbed with one to two drops of essential oils.

Room spray. Spray a room with essential oils mixed in water, fifteen to thirty drops per eight ounces of water. Shake vigorously before each use.

Baths

Baths are especially beneficial because they combine the healing effects of water (hydrotherapy) with essential oils (aromatherapy). They are helpful for muscle discomfort, skin conditions, and emotional imbalance. Fill the bathtub with warm water, immerse yourself, and then add eight to ten drops of essential oil(s). Stir the water around you and soak for ten to fifteen minutes. To relieve muscle tension use eucalyptus, or sweet marjoram; to soothe the skin use lavender, chamomile, or rose; and to relax and relieve stress use lavender, ylang ylang, clary sage, or chamomile. If there is not time for a full bath or it is inconvenient, use four drops of the same oils in a foot bath.

Massage

Massage is considered, by many, to be the best and most effective method of using essential oils for aroma-therapeutic purposes. It is gentle and rhythmic, combining the beneficial effects of touch with the properties of essential oils. Massage relaxes the muscles, and improves muscle tone, circulation, and lymph flow. It also helps release physical tension which, in turn, relieves mental stress. To make a massage oil, dilute the essential oils in canola, safflower, sweet almond, or a blend of emollient vegetable oils. A fragrance-free lotion can also be used. Standard dilution is two percent, using twenty to twenty-five drops for every two ounces of carrier oil or lotion. If the skin is very sensitive, reduce this amount to ten drops or less.

Compress

35

An aromatherapy compress is a damp, folded cloth that has been infused with essential oils and then applied to the skin, anywhere on the body. Either warm or cool water is used. Warm sedates and relaxes while cool invigorates and stimulates. In a basin of water, put two to five drops of essential oil(s). Stir briskly then lay a clean cloth (a diaper or washcloth work best) in the water, wring, and apply.

Body Splash or Mister

Mix fifteen to thirty drops of essential oil(s) in eight ounces of water, and use on the body as a splash or put in a mister. Shake well before using.

Essential Oil Safety

Because essential oils are concentrated, therapeutically-active medicinals, they can cause a physiological response, and care must be taken with their use. In many cases, it is the dilution of the essential oil that determines whether or not it can be safely used. For example, ginger can irritate the skin if used in high amount, such as five percent in a base oil. However, in low amounts, such as one percent, it can be safely used to relieve muscle aches and fatigue. Some oils, mostly citrus, can cause photosensitivity, and cannot be worn undiluted in direct sunlight. In addition to the wide range of safe and effective oils, such as frankincense, rosewood, or sandalwood, there are also a few oils that are not recommended for unsupervised, home use. These include mugwort, sassafras, thuja, pennyroyal, tansy, and others. We suggest obtaining one of the books listed in Recommended Reading at the end of this chapter to use as a reference for essential oil safety.

Note: In the context of subtle energy therapy, the amount of essential oils in a carrier oil is very low, usually at one-half percent or less. This is believed to be low enough as to not affect the physical body, instead, affecting only the subtle bodies with the oil's vibrational properties.

The following are standard, recommended safety guidelines for using essential oils:

- Do not take essential oils internally.
- Keep essential oils tightly closed and away from children.
- Keep essential oils away from and out of your eyes. (If this should occur, first put a drop of carrier oil such as canola, sweet almond, or sunflower oil in your eye to collect the essential oil. If no carrier oil is available, rinse extremely well with water.)
- Most essential oils should be diluted before they are applied to the skin.
- Citrus oils can cause sensitivity and discoloration of the skin when exposed to direct sunlight.
- If you are allergy prone, test the oil under a bandage for 12 hours. If there is no reaction, the oil should be safe to use. If there is swelling or irritation, do not use the oil.
- If you are pregnant, there are many oils you should not use. Use a reference book.
- If you have a heart condition, there are oils you should not use. Use a reference book.
- If you are taking homeopathics, essential oils may negate their effect. Check with your physician.

- Don't put essential oils near a flame. They are flammable.
- If you have epilepsy, do not use essential oils without consulting your physician.
- If you have asthma, do not inhale essential oils without medical direction.
- If your skin becomes irritated with essential oils, rub the area with a carrier oil, and discontinue use.

Aromatherapy Resources

Essential Oils

There are many excellent aromatherapy companies that offer therapeutic-quality essential oils. Inquire about them at the schools in the Education section below. The authors use oils from a variety of sources, and particularly recommend those that have not been exposed to electromagnetic machinery which can disrupt the subtle properties. The following companies take these protective measures.

Oshadhi USA
1340-G Industrial Avenue
Petaluma, CA
(707) 763-0662

Fragrant Earth
2000 2nd Avenue #206
Seattle, WA 98121
(206) 374-8773

Education
Light-Touched™
Ruah Bull and Joni Keim Loughran
On-going classes and workshops focusing on aromatherapy and subtle energy techniques for lay persons, and professional body workers and healers. Call or write for information, products, or to request a newsletter.
P.O. Box 750986
Petaluma, CA 94975-0986
(707) 573-6071
www.light-touched.com

Joni Keim Loughran
On-going introductory classes on a variety of aromatherapy
topics such as stress relief, skin care, seasonal applications,
and blending. Seminars available for professional massage
therapists, cosmetologists, and aestheticians.
(707) 765-6986

Center for Phyto-Aromatherapy
Dr. Malte Hozzel
Orto de Prouvènço
F-84390 Aurel en Provence, France
+33-4-90641378
Email: phyto-mc@imcn.com

Jeanne Rose Aromatherapy
Lectures and Seminars
219 Carl Street
San Francisco, CA 94117
(415) 564-6785

Aromatherapy Institute and Research (AIR)
Victoria Edwards
P.O. Box 2354
Fair Oaks, CA 95628
(916) 965-7546

Pacific Institute of Aromatherapy
Kurt Schnaubelt
P.O. Box 6723
San Rafael, CA 94903
(415) 479-9121

Aroma Studio
Kathy Jenkins
(888) 432-0292
(914) 651-1225
www.aromastudio.com

Michael Scholes School of Aromatic Studies
4218 N. Glencoe #4
Marina Del Rey, CA 90292
(310) 827-7737

Twin Lakes College of the Healing Arts
Aromatherapy Program
1210 Brommer Street
Santa Cruz, CA 95062
(831) 476-2152

The Foundation for Aromatherapy Research & Education
1900-C West Stone Avenue
Fairfield, IA 52556
(515) 472-9136

The College of Botanical Healing Arts
1821 17th Avenue
Santa Cruz, CA 95062
(831) 462-1807

Artemis Institute of Natural Therapies
P.O. Box 1846
Boulder, CO 80306
(303) 443-9289

The Institute of Dynamic Aromatherapy
2000 2nd Avenue #206
Seattle, WA 98121
(206) 374-8773

Associations
National Association for Holistic Aromatherapy
P.O. Box 17622
Boulder, CO 80308
(888) ASK-NAHA

Canadian Federation of Aromatherapists
439 Wellington Street West
Toronto, Ontario M5V 1E7

41

Publications
The Aromatherapy Journal (formerly Scentsitivity)
Quarterly Journal of NAHA
P.O. Box 17622
Boulder, CO 80308
(888) ASK-NAHA

Recommended Reading

The Illustrated Encyclopedia of Essential Oils, Julia Lawless (Rockport, Massachusetts: Element Books, 1995).

The Healing Power of Aromatherapy, Hasnain Walji, Ph.D. (Rocklin, California: Prima Publishing, 1996).

Aromatherapy: A Complete Guide to the Healing Art, Kathi Keville and Mindy Green (Freedom, California: The Crossing Press, 1995).

Aromatherapy For Vibrant Health and Beauty, Roberta Wilson (Garden City Park, New York: Avery Publishing Group, 1995).

Aromatherapy: A Lifetime Guide to Healing with Essential Oils, Valerie Gennari Cooksley (Englewood Cliffs, New Jersey: Prentice Hall, 1996).

The World of Aromatherapy, Edited by Jeanne Rose and Susan Earle (Berkeley, California: Frog, Ltd., 1996).

THREE

The Subtle Properties of Essential Oils

We have discussed aromatherapy and the nature of essential oils, explaining how they affect us wholistically—physically, psychologically, and energetically. Now, we will explore in more detail, their energetic qualities.

What is Vibrational Medicine?

Vibrational medicine is a term often used to describe the variety of modalities that influence the energy centers and subtle bodies. Subtle energy therapy using hands and subtle aromatherapy are both types of vibrational medicine, belonging to a group of therapies that are perceived and interpreted by our sensory organs on one level and our energy field on another. Subtle energy therapy using hands relates to our sense of touch and subtle aromatherapy to our sense of smell. The other senses, sight, sound, and taste, also have corresponding modalities—color therapy, music therapy, and taste therapy. Beyond our senses, well known examples of vibrational medicine are homeopathy and flower essence therapy.

Patricia Davis, in *Subtle Aromatherapy,* describes the principle behind the effectiveness of vibrational medicine, "Nothing in the universe is still . . . If we look at the body in the most minute detail every one of its millions of cells vibrates with its own life pattern." Describing the exquisite harmony in the movement of cells, she explains, "This harmony is both a reflection of the cell's health and the source of that health, for as long as the cell moves in its ordered dance every function of that cell will take place in an orderly way, and we experience this as a state of health."

If the order breaks down, the function of the cell is disturbed, and physical or psychological imbalance can follow. Therefore, the goal of

45

vibrational therapy is to restore erratic cellular vibration to its original, healthy pattern by *persuasive resonance*—that is, by gently coaxing it to mirror the optimal vibrational model. Note: The correction of cellular vibration assists in correcting the imbalance of corresponding energy centers.

How the Subtle Properties of Essential Oils are Determined

The subtle or vibrational properties of essential oils are used for the purpose of influencing cellular vibration, as described above. When the chemical constituents of an essential oil are analyzed, the results determine the physical application of the essential oil, such as anti-inflammatory, expectorant, or anti-bacterial. Chemical analysis alone cannot be used to ascertain the subtle or vibrational properties. Instead, they are learned from evaluating the long-term, traditional uses of both the essential oil and herb of the same plant, the physical and psychological affects of the oil, the gesture and signature of the plant itself (its appearance and characteristics), and from personal experience.

46

The aromatic qualities of plants have been used for religious ritual, meditation, and prayer for thousands of years. Fragrances were chosen for

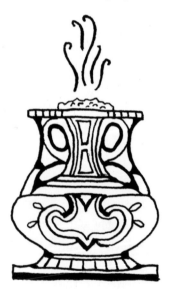

their ability to promote feelings of oneness with the universe, and a closeness with God. These spiritual connections have been passed down through the ages from ancient Egypt, Arabia, Greece, and Asia, as well as other cultures such as native American. Dried herbs were burned as incense, and the rising smoke was believed to communicate with the deities. As it rose to the heavens, prayers were offered. Frankincense was the most common aromatic used, and is mentioned several times in the Bible, most notably as a gift to baby Jesus. Sage was traditionally used by native Americans in ceremony.

The known physical and psychological effects of essential oils are often indicators of their subtle properties. For example, rosemary promotes mental clarity and relieves mental fatigue. On a subtle level, rosemary has an affinity with the sixth energy center (Third Eye), and is used to promote clear thoughts and insight. On a physical level, juniper is cleansing and antiseptic. On a subtle level, it is used to cleanse a room of negativity, and to detoxify the subtle bodies.

Plant gestures and signatures are how the plant expresses itself—a representation of transformed energy from the sun and the earth. These gestures and signatures are used to help determine flower essence properties, and are useful to determine essential oil subtle properties as well. Look at the plant (or its picture) from which the essential oil comes. What is it trying to say? Note its color or the color of its essential oil. Record where it grows, its fragrance, and its size. Does it look hardy or fragile? Is it tall or short? The plant's appearance and character is an indication of what it will offer in the subtle realm. For example, blue chamomile calms and reduces inflammation. On a subtle level, it works on the fifth energy center (Throat) which vibrates to the color blue, quieting angry words and promoting calm, clear communication.

Malte Hozzel, an internationally known naturalist and essential oil specialist, has a unique understanding and appreciation of the plant kingdom. In this passage, he compares the gestures of two plants from which essential oils are extracted, clary sage and true sage. "Look at the huge, green leaves and the thick stem of the clary sage with her large mauve and pink blossoms. Clary is incarnated nature, fully there, expansive and strong. It's scent is musky, sweet, and floral. Everything tells us about a balance between material and ethereal forces. It has powerful harmonizing and euphorizing qualities, combining in rare beauty both earthly and celestial energies. On the other hand, the true sage has a thin stem and small, purple-violet blossoms. Its fragrance is warm, fresh and herbaceous. It has iridescent, fine, greyish-blue hairs on the surface of its small and soft leaves. Everything tells us about refinement, subtlety. The life force seems to be

47

drawn towards another dimension. Its subtle, vibrational energies work in true correspondence with the finer energies of our central nervous system."

Last, and most important, is personal experience, including information received intuitively. Because essential oils are used energetically with intent, their purpose can be designed, directed, and influenced. For example, rose is an essential oil that promotes love and has a strong affinity with the Heart center. However, it can be used with intent on the Third Eye to assist one in experiencing loving thoughts. It might be used on the Root center to encourage love of life. As you work more with essential oils in subtle energy therapy, you may have experiences that indicate a different property than known or described in this book. You may have a strong feeling that an oil is not working the way it should, or that a certain oil is working differently or better than has been indicated. It is possible for this to happen, so it is important to trust your responses and instincts. However, it is also important to get feedback from your receiver. If you choose to use an unfamiliar oil, or want to learn more about a favorite oil, try the following exercise.

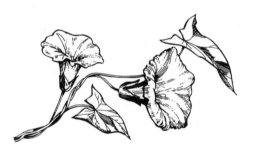

Listening to the Oils

"Listening to the Oils" is one method that the authors use to understand an essential oil and its subtle application. When working with and exploring subtle properties, it is helpful for you to learn how to use your feelings and intuition to gather vital information. This exercise will help you to relax, focus, and "listen" while an essential oil communicates with you, especially when experiencing the oil for the first time.

Pick an oil you would like to explore, and place the bottle near you.

Find a quiet place where you will be undisturbed for about 20 minutes.

Settle into a comfortable position with your back supported. If, during this process, you need to change position, it will not interfere with your internal focus.

Take a few, deep, relaxing breaths, and follow these steps:

At the count of 1, take a deep breath and lift your eyes to look up at your eyebrows.

At the count of 2, exhale and close your eyes.

At the count of 3, repeat a few relaxing words to yourself as you inhale, such as, "Relax, release, let go."

At the count of 4, release the breath with an audible sigh and imagine a beautiful wave of relaxation pouring into your crown energy center, filling your body with a wonderful sense of calm, as you keep breathing. When your body is full, imagine that the energy centers on the bottoms of your feet open, and any remaining stress, tension, or negativity flows out of your body as naturally as water running down a drain. Then imagine those centers closing to their normal size. Take a moment to enjoy this experience.

In this relaxed state, you will be in close contact with your intuitive mind, and you can invite your rational mind to observe the following process.

When you are ready, pick up the bottle of oil you have chosen to explore, and hold it in your hands for a moment to perceive its vibrational quality. Notice any impressions you receive as you hold it. You may sense a color, experience a feeling, or recall a memory. You may detect a texture, or an image may appear to you. Some people hear sounds or music. Some

49

smell a fragrance which may or may not be the fragrance of the oil. Jot down any of your impressions on a piece of paper. You may not receive any impression at all. Remember, there is no right or wrong way for this process—we each experience impressions in our own way, in our own time.

Now open the bottle, put a drop on a tissue, and smell it, letting the fragrance fill you.

With your eyes closed, become aware of the fragrance, and notice any impressions you receive. (You may smell the oil more than once, but not too frequently.) Do you like or dislike the aroma? Are there any places in your body that react or feel affected by this fragrance? Is there an energy center that is touched or stimulated? Does it make you feel relaxed or energized? Do you receive any sense impressions such as a color, shape, temperature or texture? Do you see an image, hear a sound, or recall a memory? Without forcing a judgement, notice any impressions, and write them down.

50

Now imagine you are engaged in a conversation with this oil. Ask the following questions, and write down your responses. Your responses may come in any sense—as words, feelings, images, or sounds. Ask the oil:

What are your subtle properties?

Complete this statement: "I am _____."

With what energy center are you most connected?

What are your energy gifts?

What are your spiritual gifts?

Is there anything about you that you want me to know?

Is there anything you want to communicate to me now?

Ask any other question(s) that are meaningful for you.

This exercise may seem unusual, but it is quite helpful in assisting your intuition to receive information from the energetic properties of an essential oil. The more you practice, the easier, and more natural it will be.

When you have finished with the oil, be grateful for its willingness to communicate with you in this way.

Take a few, deep breaths, and count backwards from 4 to return to ordinary consciousness: 4, take a slow, deep breath; 3, be aware of your body and the room; 2, wiggle your fingers and toes with another deep breath; and 1, feel awake, alert, and refreshed.

Now you have completed the intuitive aspect of listening to the oils. When you begin using the oils in a subtle energy session, always ask for feedback from your receiver. Be aware that intuitive insights need to be substantiated in experiment and experience. If you are working with an oil, and it doesn't seem to be doing what you expected, go back and listen further for more information or clarification. You can begin to communicate and connect with essential oils just as you would with any trusted companion. For your convenience, Appendix III is a form that can be photocopied and used for this exercise.

The Subtle Properties of Essential Oils: A-Z

Most essential oils have numerous applications in subtle energy therapy. For example, sandalwood is grounding when used with the first energy center, it increases sexual energy when used with the second, and encourages states of higher consciousness used with the seventh. Following is a list of essential oils, their perceived subtle properties, and their correlating energy center. Keep in mind that these properties are supported, influenced, and directed by intent, which is further discussed in Chapter 4.

Ammi visnaga (*Ammi visnaga*)

SIXTH: Supports the development of intuition by increasing the energy in the left brain. Increases the ability to creatively visualize. Brings clarity and objectivity to intuitive information.

Amyris (*Amyris balsamifera*)

SIXTH: Supports the development of the right brain to increase creativity.

Angelica Root (*Angelica archangelica*)

FIRST: Grounds.

SIXTH AND SEVENTH: Connects us with angelic guidance. Encourages the presence of angels. Strengthens the spirit. Aligns us with our higher selves. Balances and protects us during meditative, healing states.

Anise (*Pimpinella anisum*)

GENERAL: Clears and cleanses the auric field so that energy can move easily through the various subtle bodies.

SIXTH AND SEVENTH: Clears and cleanses these centers of old thought forms so that spiritual information can be received.

Artemisia (*Artemisia afra*)

FIRST AND SECOND: Helps us to fully connect and embrace the earthly experience. Good for people who think that being spiritual means rejecting the world.

52

Azalea absolute (Azalea)
GENERAL: Helps to integrate masculine and feminine energies.
SEVENTH: Releases emotions lodged in the astral subtle body that interfere with receiving spiritual guidance, and prevents us from knowing our spiritual path.

Basil (Ocimum basilicum)
GENERAL: Uplifts the spirits.
SIXTH: Clears the mind.

Bay Laurel (Laurus nobilis)
SIXTH: Promotes psychic awareness and intuition. Provides psychic protection. Opens us to new thoughts and perspectives. Releases mental blocks and outmoded ways of thinking.

Benzoin (Styrax benzoin)
GENERAL: Dispels anger and negativity.
FIRST: Grounds and comforts.
SIXTH: Provides psychic protection. Steadies and focuses the mind for meditation or prayer. Allows buried thoughts and feelings to come safely to consciousness to be examined and processed.

Bergamot (Citrus bergamia)
GENERAL: Brings in positive energy.
FIRST: Supports love of our physical body.
FOURTH: Supports self-love. Opens the Heart center and allows love to radiate. Eases grief.

Birch (Betula alba)
GENERAL: Clears and cleanses. Releases fear.
THIRD: Promotes courage.

Black pepper (Piper nigrum)
GENERAL: Dissolves energy blockages caused by anger and frustration.
THIRD: Increases courage.

Broom absolute (Spartium junceum)
FIRST: Helps to ground people who are too much "in their heads."
SEVENTH: Brings spiritual sustenance to people over-attached to the material world.

Bucco leaves (Barosma buchulina)
FIRST: Assists grounding under any circumstances.

Cabreuva (Myrocarpus fastigiatus)
GENERAL: Brings all of the energy centers into balance and harmony with each other while it clears and cleanses. Seals and protects the auric field to promote healthy boundaries.

Cajeput (Melaleuca cajeputi)
GENERAL: Connects us with child-like devotion and trust in the universe.

Calamus (Acorus calamus)
GENERAL: Good for any kind of spiritual/intuitive work. Brings information directly from the Seventh center so that it can be clearly understood by the mind (Sixth center) and communicated effectively (Fifth).

Cardamom (Ellettaria cardamomum)
GENERAL: Helps to teach others with a grounded, clear, heart-centered perspective.
FIRST: Helps us to accept life as it is while encouraging an enthusiasm for it.
SECOND: Stimulates sexual energy.
SIXTH: Clears the conscious mind.

Carvi (Carum carvi)
FIFTH: A superb oil to assist with all issues related to this center. Promotes clear communication and good listening.

Cascarilla (Croton niveous)
THIRD CENTER: Promotes personal will, integrity, and healthy self-esteem.

54

Cedarwood (Cedrus atlantica)
GENERAL: Clears and cleanses a room. Brings in positive energy.
FIRST: Connects us with earthly forces. Grounds.
THIRD: Strengthens confidence and will.
SIXTH: Clears and steadies the mind. Promotes a calm meditative state to better receive healing energy.
SEVENTH: Restores a sense of spiritual certainty. Strengthens the connection with the divine.

Cedrella (Cedrella odorata)
THIRD CENTER: Acts as a general tonic. Clears and cleanses to release any negative energy while promoting healthy self-esteem, will power, and integrity.

Chamomile, German (Chamomila matricaria)
GENERAL: Calms. Balances emotions.
FIFTH: Supports the calm, clear speaking of our truth.

Chamomile, Roman (Anthemis nobilis)
GENERAL: Calms. Balances emotions.
THIRD: Calm acceptance of our own limitations. Eases the tensions associated with excessive ego such as frustration and resentment. Promotes patience.
FOURTH: Eases grief and sadness.
FIFTH AND SEVENTH: Connects these two centers to facilitate hearing and communicating our spiritual truth.

Champaca (Michelia champaca)
GENERAL: Energizes and balances the auric field and energy centers.
THIRD, FOURTH, FIFTH, SIXTH, AND SEVENTH CENTERS: Assists these centers, as a group, to move to a higher level of spiritual development.
SIXTH: Opens the mind to the influx of Divine energy and information. Assists psychic development.

55

Cinnamon, leaf (Cinnamomum verum)
GENERAL: Strengthens.
SIXTH: Increases psychic abilities. Helps recover memories.

Cistus (Cistus ladaniferus)
SIXTH AND SEVENTH: Assists in receiving clear messages from spiritual guides.

Citronella (Cymbopogon winterianus)
FIRST THROUGH FIFTH: Connects and balances these energy centers, bringing the lower centers (First through Fourth) into alignment with Divine will.

Clary sage (Salvia sclarea)
GENERAL: Calms and uplifts.
SIXTH: Increases dreaming. Strengthens our inner eye to "see" more clearly. Inspires.

Clove (Eugenia caryophyllata)
GENERAL: Supports the process of releasing outmoded thoughts and feelings.
THIRD: Heightens courage.
SIXTH: Strengthens the conscious mind. Assists in recovering memories.

Costus root (Saussurea lappa)
GENERAL: Balances all the energy centers. Balances and cleanses the etheric body to provide the healthiest possible blueprint for the physical body. Good for grounding after meditation.

Croton anisatum (Croton anisatum)
GENERAL: Clears and balances negative emotions, such as fear, anger, and greed so that actions can be taken from a calm, centered awareness.

Copaiva balm (Copaifera reticulata)
SIXTH AND SEVENTH: Connects these two energy centers, aligning the human mind with the spiritual mind.

Coriander (Coriandrum sativum)
General: Speeds the healing process.
First: Promotes feelings of security.
Second: Increases creativity, spontaneity, and passion.
Third: Promotes confidence and motivation.
Sixth: Improves memory.

Curry leaves (Murraya koenigii)
Seventh: Helps in spiritual evolution. Opens us to divine energy and guidance.

Cypress (Cupressus sempervirens)
General: Strengthens and comforts. Assists in times of transition. Supports willingness to change and transform.
Third: Promotes confidence and patience.
Sixth: Promotes wisdom.

Cypriol (Cyperus scariosus)
General: Helps to find a positive perspective in hard times and situations.
Sixth: Helps to see clearly when experiencing difficult emotions.

Dill (Anethum graveolens)
General: Clears a room of negative emotional energies such as anger, fear, or jealousy.

Elecampane (Inula helenium)
General: Excellent for clearing the astral level of the subtle bodies. Seals and protects the astral body.
Second: Assists in balancing all the issues related to this center—creativity, emotions, and sexuality. Provides protection.

Elemi (Canarium luzonicum)
First: Grounds after deep meditation. Balances the spiritual and worldly life.
Sixth and Seventh: Opens us to mystical experiences. Balances the spiritual and worldly life.

57

Erigeron (Conyza canadensis)
General: Helps in discovering one's life purpose.
Sixth and Seventh: Opens these centers to allow spiritual energy to enter.

Eriocephalus (Eriocephalus africanus)
General: Good after meditation to both ground and assist the integration of information. Helps us to slow down mentally and physically so we can be more spiritually attuned. Balances and grounds.

Eucalyptus (Eucalyptus radiata)
General: Clears and cleanses a room. Dissolves energy blockages. Balances emotions.
Fourth: Promotes room to breathe when feeling disheartened and suffocated by responsibilities.
Sixth: Inspires. Promotes concentration.

Fennel (Foeniculum vulgare)
General: Provides protection from negative, psychic influences.
Third: Increases courage, confidence, and motivation.
Fifth: Promotes uninhibited communication.

Fir, Silver (Abies alba)
General: Releases energy blocks. Balances emotions.
First: Grounds.
Sixth: Increases intuition.

Fokienia (Fokienia hodginsii)
General: Promotes courage and clarity during times of stress. Balances and grounds all the energy centers to promote the development of courage, integrity, focus, purpose, and compassion.

Frangipani (Plumeria rubia)

GENERAL: Promotes healing in our relationship with our mother. Helps us to expand our capacity to nurture others.

FIRST: Helps to heal our relationship with Mother Earth. Helps spiritual people embrace and love the earthly experience.

SEVENTH: Promotes an awareness of the feminine aspect of the Divine.

Frankincense (Boswellia carterii)

GENERAL: Calms, comforts, and centers. Stabilizes emotions.

FIRST: Grounds.

SIXTH: Quiets and clarifies the mind. Promotes a meditative state to better receive and integrate healing energy.

SEVENTH: Focuses and strengthens spiritual consciousness and enlightenment. Connects us with the eternal and Divine.

Galbanum (Ferula galbaniflua)

SEVENTH: Connects us with Divine trust and innocence.

Galgant Root (Alpinia Galanga)

THIRD: Helps the personal will to become healthy, clear, and balanced. Develops personal integrity.

Geranium (Pelargonium graveolens)

GENERAL: Calms the mind and spirit. Promotes harmony and happiness in relationships. Balances the emotions.

SECOND: Fosters creativity and sensory experience. Nourishes feminine creativity. Promotes relaxed spontaneity.

THIRD: Helps us to gain control of our lives.

FIFTH: Increases capacity for intimate communication.

SEVENTH: Provides spiritual protection.

59

Ginger (Zingiber officinalis)
GENERAL: Strengthens.
SECOND: Increases sexual desire.
THIRD: Promotes courage and confidence.

Gingerlily (Hedychium spicatum)
FOURTH: Strengthens the heart energetically to be able to physically and mentally experience more love. Increases compassion.

Golden Rod (Solidago canadensis)
GENERAL: Encourages the influence of spiritual guidance.
FIFTH: Helps to balance this center so that listening and communication improves.

Grapefruit (Citrus paradisii)
GENERAL: Dissolves emotional energy blocks especially frustration and self-blame.
THIRD: Promotes confidence.
SIXTH: Increases intuition and mental clarity. Inspires.

Greenland Moss (Ledum groenlandicum)
GENERAL: Increases memory and clarity of thought. Encourages left brain rationality for projects imagined by the intuitive right brain.
SEVENTH: Encourages balanced spiritual energy.

Guaiac Wood (Bulnesia sarmienti)
GENERAL: Balances and heals all the energy centers so that a person can walk their spiritual path with clarity and integrity. Assists in finding one's life work and purpose.
THIRD AND SEVENTH: Encourages spirituality to influence personal will. Helps to prepare the personality for spiritual development.

Gurjum (Dipteropcarpus turbinatua)
GENERAL: Supports meditative states. Activates the intuitive mind.
SIXTH AND SEVENTH: Helps to open these centers to receive spiritual energy.

Hay (Foenum)
GENERAL: Helps with meditation. Helps to connect with intuitive guidance, especially from the plant kingdom.

Hyssop (Hyssopus officinalis decumbens)
GENERAL: Clears negative energy.
THIRD: Provides protection from others' moods and emotions. Eases feelings of guilt.
FOURTH: Eases feelings of grief.
SEVENTH: Heightens spirituality.

Immortelle (Helichrysum angustifolium)
GENERAL: Dissolves energy blockages. Balances the upper energy centers.
FOURTH: Promotes compassion for self and others. Integrates compassion and spirituality.
SIXTH: Activates the right side of the brain. Assists in communicating psychic impressions. Promotes understanding.

Jasmine (Jasminum officinale)
GENERAL: Unites and harmonizes opposites to promote wholeness. Calms, soothes, relaxes, and lifts the spirits. Releases worry to allow living in the present moment.
SECOND: Promotes love and sensuality. Connects spirituality and sexuality. Promotes creativity and artistic development.
FOURTH: Warms and opens the heart.
SIXTH: Enhances intuition. Opens the mind to deeper truths. Inspires.
SEVENTH: Connects spirituality and sexuality. Heightens spiritual awareness.

61

Juniper (Juniperus communis)

GENERAL: Clears and cleanses a room of negative energies. Protects against negative influences. Clears energetic blockages. Cleanses and detoxifies the subtle bodies.

THIRD: Strengthens will power and eases fear of failure, restoring confidence and increasing self-worth.

SIXTH: Dispels mental stagnation. Assists clairvoyance if used for altruistic reasons. Promotes inner vision and wisdom.

SEVENTH: Helps us to connect with and act from our highest ideals. Enlightens.

Kanuka (Leptospermum ericoides)

GENERAL: Balances all the energy centers. Increases feelings of joy.

Lantana (Lantana camara)

FIFTH: Promotes the gift of hearing guidance (clairaudience). Helps to develop awareness of our own inner voice.

Larch (Larix laricina)

GENERAL: Promotes clarity of thoughts and feelings. Energizes and uplifts.

Lavender (Lavendula vera)

GENERAL: One of the most important subtle energy oils. Balances all energy centers and subtle bodies. Useful in all energy healing techniques to relax and balance. Clears and cleanses a room. Brings in positive energy.

FOURTH: Calms, comforts, and stabilizes emotions of the heart. Promotes compassion.

SEVENTH: Helps to integrate spirituality in everyday life. Promotes spiritual growth.

HANDS: Increases awareness and sensitivity to healing energy work.

Lemon (Citrus limonum)

GENERAL: Clears and cleanses the room. Clears emotional confusion and invigorates.

FOURTH: Helps to alleviate fears of emotional involvement. Promotes joy.

SIXTH: Promotes objectivity and mental clarity. Focuses consciousness.

Lemongrass (Cympobogon citratus)
GENERAL: Clears and cleanses the room. Dispels negative energy.
SIXTH: Stimulates psychic awareness.

Leptospermum (Leptospermum citratum)
SIXTH: Assists the modern person to understand and integrate the ancient wisdom of indigenous people.

Lime (Citrus aurantifolia)
GENERAL: Clears and cleanses the room. Purifies the mind and body.
SIXTH: Provides psychic protection.

Lovage (Levisticum officinale)
FIRST: Grounds and centers. Opens the Base and feet energy centers to receive earth energy.
HANDS: Opens hand centers so that healing earth energy can be sent to the receiver easily and without draining the giver's energy.

Magnolia (Magnolia grandiflora)
FOURTH: Increases the ability to give and receive love.
FIFTH: Increases the ability to speak about and hear love.

Mandarin (Citrus reticulata)
GENERAL: Promotes joy and happiness.
FIFTH: Promotes communication with the inner child.
SIXTH: Inspires.

Mangoginger (Cureuma amada)
SECOND: Promotes playful sensuality. Reduces fear and other effects of emotional and physical traumas pertaining to sexuality. Promotes sexual joy.

Marjoram (Origanum majorana)
GENERAL: Comforts. Reduces fear.
FIRST: Comforts and supports.
THIRD: Promotes confidence and courage.
FOURTH: Helps us to accept deep, emotional loss. Promotes ability to give.
SIXTH: Unifies the right and left brain.

63

Mastic (Pistacia lentiscus)
General: Increases our physical energy to allow for greater spiritual energy.
Seventh: Creates a direct and immediate connection with Divine guidance.

Meadowsweet (Filipendula ulmaria)
General: Connects us with the angelic realm.

Meerfenchel (Cribimum maritimum)
General: Helps us to deal with challenging situations with strength and focus.
Third: The "cloak of power." Promotes a sense of personal power and protection.

Melissa (Melissa officinalis)
General: Helps to deal with issues about death. Promotes emotional clarity. Promotes understanding and acceptance.
Fourth: Relieves emotional blocks due to grief.
Seventh: Promotes spiritual growth.

Mimosa (Acacia dealbata)
Fourth: Opens the heart to receive love.
Sixth: Promotes psychic dreams.

Monarda (Monarda didyma)
Seventh: A spiritual gatekeeper that allows us to perceive, receive or understand information for which we are ready. Prevents spiritual confusion and feeling overwhelmed.

Myrrh (Commiphora myrrha)
General: Strengthens and energizes. Supports earthy manifestations of dreams and visions by linking higher energy centers with the Base energy center.
First: Grounds during meditation.
Fourth: Eases sorrow and grief.
Fifth: Provides support for confident communication.
Sixth: Grounds during meditation.
Seventh: Assists in moving forward on our spiritual journey. Fortifies spirituality.

64

Myrtle (Myrtus communis)
GENERAL: Provides protection during major life transitions. Promotes harmony, love, and respect.
SEVENTH: Supports connections with angels.

Narcissus (Narcissus poeticus)
SECOND: Promotes creativity.
FOURTH: Eases grief and hopelessness. Helps to heal emotional wounds.
SIXTH: Inspires. Increases inner visions.

Neroli (Citrus aurantium)
GENERAL: Brings in positive energy. Relaxes. Helps us face our emotional fears. Links lower and higher selves—soul and spirit.
SECOND: Promotes sensual comfort.
FOURTH: Eases grief. Helps us experience joyful love.
SIXTH: Reunites the conscious and subconscious minds.
SEVENTH: Promotes direct communication with the spiritual world.

Niaouli (Melaleuca quinquenervia)
SIXTH: Protects against negative, psychic influences.

Nigella Seeds (Nigella sativa)
GENERAL: Grounds, balances, protects, and enhances all the centers.

Nutmeg (Myristica fragrans)
SECOND: Increases creativity.
SIXTH: Increases psychic abilities and creativity.

Oakmoss (Evernia prunastri)
FIRST: Grounds during spiritual journey work. Increases sense of prosperity and security.

Opopanax (Commiphora erythraea)
GENERAL: Helps to heal physical, emotional, mental, and spiritual wounds. Provides physical and psychic protection.
SIXTH: Opens us to mystical understanding.

65

Orange (Citrus aurantium)
GENERAL: Brings in positive energy. Nourishes the soul with joy. Moves stagnated energy.
SECOND: Promotes joy in sexuality and creativity.
THIRD: Promotes self-confidence and courage.
FOURTH: Promotes joyful love.

Palmarosa (Cympobogon martinii)
GENERAL: Aids in all types of healing—physical, emotional, mental, and spiritual. Diffuse in the room to speed the body's ability to heal.
FIRST: Encourages feelings of security.
FOURTH: Comforts the heart.
SIXTH: Clears the mind to help with decision-making. Develops wisdom.

Pastinak (Pastinaca sativa)
SIXTH: Supports the left brain to bring in the best qualities of "common sense"—clear, calm, grounded, practical, logical.

66

Patchouli (Pogostemon patchouli)
GENERAL: Grounds and soothes.
FIRST: Strengthens and grounds, relieving deficiencies in Base energy center. Re-attaches the physical body with subtle bodies.
SECOND: Spiritualizes sexuality. Facilitates enjoyment of the senses and awakening of creativity.
SIXTH: Relaxes a tense, over-active intellect.
FEET CENTERS: Opens feet centers to connect with and draw earth energy.

Peppermint (Mentha piperita)
GENERAL: Clarifies.
THIRD: Promotes healthy self-esteem, integrity, and ethics. Helps us discover our hidden gifts and strengths.
FIFTH: Promotes clarity in communication and concentration.
SIXTH: Calms nerves while it stimulates the conscious mind. Promotes inspiration and insights.

Peru Balsam (Myroxylon balsamum)
FIRST: Promotes feelings of safety and of being nurtured.
SECOND: Promotes sensuality and confidence.

Petitgrain (Citrus aurantium)
GENERAL: Brings in positive energy. Promotes optimism.
THIRD: Promotes a healthy self-esteem and trust in self and others.
SIXTH: Stimulates the conscious mind and clears perception. Increases inner visions.

Pine (Pinus sylvestris)
GENERAL: Clears and cleanses a room. Repels and clears negative energy. Increases energy in the subtle bodies. Useful for anyone who is depleted or feeling stagnant.
THIRD: Restores self-confidence and strength of will.

Rose (Rosa damascena)
GENERAL: Brings in positive energy. Gently fills auric holes and seals the auric field after healing work. Promotes a sense of well-being.
SECOND: Connects sexuality with the Heart center. Promotes creativity and love of beauty.
FOURTH: Promotes love, compassion, hope, and patience. Calms and supports the Heart center. Heals emotional wounds, especially grief.
SEVENTH: Promotes a sense of spiritual connection and completeness.
HAND CENTERS: Connects the hands to the heart, energetically.

Rosemary (Rosmarinus officinalis)
GENERAL: Clears and cleanses a room. Provides protection from negative influences. Helps to establish healthy boundaries in relationships. Strengthens and centers.
THIRD: Promotes self-confidence. Promotes action. Strengthens will power.
FOURTH: Inspires joyful love.
SIXTH: Clears the mind. Enhances memory. Provides psychic protection. Promotes clear thoughts, insights, and understanding.
SEVENTH: Helps us to remember our spiritual path. Inspires faith.

67

Rosewood (*Aniba roseodora*)

GENERAL: Brings in positive energy. Dissolves energy blockages.

THIRD: Promotes self-acceptance.

SEVENTH: Opens us to spirituality, gently modulating the timing of the opening.

Sandalwood (*Santalum album*)

GENERAL: Supports all healing work. Calms and comforts.

FIRST: Grounds and re-connects us with our sense of being.

SECOND: Promotes spiritual sensuality. Increases sexual energy.

THIRD: Promotes positive self-esteem.

FOURTH: Helps to open the heart to trust, and to receive healing energy.

SIXTH: Quiets the mind. Promotes a meditative state to better receive and integrate healing energy. Promotes deep meditation and wisdom.

SEVENTH: Encourages states of higher consciousness and sense of unity.

Santolina (*Santolina chamaecyparissus*)

GENERAL: Supports the feminine nature. Helps to access the innocent joy of a young woman and the experienced wisdom of maturity.

Savory, Winter (*Satureja montana*)

GENERAL: Helps us to appreciate, connect, and understand the wisdom and spirituality found in nature.

SECOND AND SEVENTH: Links these two centers, spiritualizing the emotions.

Schinus (*Schinus molle l.*)

GENERAL: Provides protection when being verbally or energetically attacked.

SIXTH: Helps us to understand and grow from the experiences of being verbally or energetically "attacked."

68

Spikenard (Nardostachys jatamansi)
GENERAL: Embodies wholeness. Promotes a sense of hope.
FOURTH: Comforts and balances the heart, especially for people who take on the cares of the world.
FIFTH: Helps communication between humans and animals.
SEVENTH: Increases love and devotion for God, higher self, and the Divine.

Spruce (Picea mariana)
GENERAL: Clears and cleanses.
FIRST: Grounds intuition so that it can be clear and practical.
FOURTH: Infuses intuition with compassion.
FIFTH: Promotes communication of inner feelings.
SIXTH: Brings objectivity and clarity to the intuitive mind. Develops intuition.

St. John's Wort (Hypericum perforatum)
SIXTH: Opens the mind to receive psychic dreams. Assists in understanding the personal meaning of dreams.

Tolu-Balsam (Myroxylon balsamum)
GENERAL: Helps us to feel that life is precious and sweet. Connects and balances all the centers.

Tarragon (Artemisia dracunculus)
GENERAL: Helps us to recognize and understand intuitive information that we experience as "gut feelings."

Tea Tree (Melaleuca alternifolia)
GENERAL: Promotes feelings of being connected to pure, life energy. Provides protection.
THIRD: Builds confidence.

69

Thyme (Thymus vulgaris linalol)
GENERAL: Relieves fear and apathy. Clears energy blockages.
THIRD: Promotes self-confidence and courage.
SIXTH: Re-orients and re-activates the left brain after a subtle energy session without hindering the deep processing that will continue in the subtle bodies. Promotes focus and concentration.
SEVENTH: Restores spiritual fortitude.

Tuberose (Polianthes tuberosa)
GENERAL: Calms and soothes strong emotions.
THIRD: Promotes motivation and enthusiasm.
FOURTH: Invites love into our lives. Expands our capability to give and receive love.
SIXTH: Encourages honest and frank communication.

Valerian (Valeriana officinalis)
FOURTH: Comforts the heart.
SEVENTH: Increases love for the Divine.

70

Vanilla (Vanilla planifolia)
FIRST: Encourages feelings of safety and comfort.
SECOND: Promotes sensuality.

Verbena (Lippia citriodora)
GENERAL: Clears and cleanses the room. Dispels negativity.
SECOND: Stimulates creativity.

Vetiver (Vetiveria zizanoides)
GENERAL: Clears and cleanses a room. Brings in positive energy. Protects the auric field. Grounds and centers. Protects against over-sensitivity.
FIRST: Calms and grounds. Promotes strength and a deep sense of belonging.
THIRD: Promotes positive self-esteem.
SIXTH: Promotes wisdom.
SEVENTH: Promotes spiritual calmness.

Violet (Viola odorata)
GENERAL: Protects those who are shy or hypersensitive.
SEVENTH: Increases spirituality.

Wormwood (Artemisia herba alba)
GENERAL: Promotes psychic dreams and increases psychic abilities. Eases times of transition.
FIRST, SECOND, THIRD: Helps us to deal with fear of death.

Yarrow, blue (Achillea millefolium)
GENERAL: Provides protection.
THIRD: Instills courage.
FOURTH: Increases healthy love for one self and others.
SIXTH: Increases and focuses psychic awareness.

Ylang Ylang (Cananga odorata)
GENERAL: Promotes feelings of peace. Dispels anger and fear.
SECOND: Increases sensuality. Helps unite our emotional and sexual natures.
THIRD: Promotes self-confidence and enthusiasm.

71

Choosing Your First Oils

There are many wonderful essential oils to use when giving a subtle energy session. The following lists are the the top twelve basic, intermediate, and advanced oils. Basic oils are indispensable and are usually the first oils you will want to have. They have many general applications and are readily accessible. The intermediate oils are a good addition to your basic set. The advanced oils have more specific purposes, and are invaluable for certain circumstances.

Your preference for particular oils will develop over time and experience. There is security in using familiar oils, and it's fun to try new ones. Enjoy the exploration.

Top 12 Basic Essential Oils

Cedarwood: Clears and cleanses a room. Brings in positive energy. Grounds.

Chamomile, Roman: Calms. Eases grief and sadness.

Eucalyptus: Clears and cleanses a room. Dissipates energy blockages.

Frankincense: Grounds. Calms. Comforts.

Lavender: Relaxes and balances. Brings in positive energy.

Lemon: Clears and cleanses a room. Promotes mental clarity.

Orange: Brings in positive energy. Promotes joy.

Peppermint: Promotes healthy self-esteem and clarity in communication.

Rose: Promotes creativity, love, compassion, joy, and a sense of well-being.

Rosemary: Clears and cleanses a room. Strengthens and centers the mind. Protects.

Sandalwood: Calms and comforts. Quiets the mind.

Vetiver: Clears and cleanses a room. Grounds. Calms. Protects.

Top 12 Intermediate Essential Oils

Benzoin: Grounds and comforts. Focuses the mind for meditation or prayer.

Chamomile, German: Calms. Promotes the calm speaking of truth.

Geranium: Balances. Calms. Promotes harmony in relationships.

Grapefruit: Disperses energy blockages. Promotes confidence.

Jasmine: Calms. Uplifts. Inspires. Promotes love, creativity, and intuition.

Juniper: Clears and cleanses a room. Protects against negativity.

Marjoram: Comforts. Promotes confidence.

Myrrh: Strengthens and supports. Grounds. Eases sorrow and grief.

Palmarosa: Comforts the heart. Supports healing on all levels.

Patchouli: Grounds. Soothes. Strengthens. Relaxes.

Rosewood: Brings in positive energy. Disperses energy blockages.

Thyme: Clears energy blockages. Promotes self-confidence, courage, and clear thinking.

Top 12 Advanced Essential Oils

Angelica: Grounds. Connects us with angelic guidance.

Bergamot: Brings in positive energy. Promotes love. Eases grief.

Champaca: Energizes and balances the auric field and energy centers.

Clary Sage: Calms. Uplifts. Inspires.

Coriander: Speeds the healing process. Promotes creativity and confidence.

Elemi: Grounds. Balances the worldly and spiritual life.

Immortelle: Disperses energy blockages. Promotes compassion.

Melissa: Promotes emotional clarity. Eases grief.

Neroli: Brings in positive energy. Eases grief.

Oakmoss: Grounds. Increases sense of prosperity and security.

Spikenard: Promotes sense of hope. Comforts the heart.

Yarrow, blue: Provides protection. Promotes courage.

73

Recommended Reading

Aromatherapy for Healing the Spirit, Gabriel Mojay (New York: Henry Holt and Company, 1996).

Subtle Aromatherapy, Patricia Davis (England: C. W. Daniels Co. Ltd., 1991).

Aromatherapy for Vibrant Health and Beauty, Roberta Wilson (Garden City Park, New York: Avery Publishing Group, 1995).

The Fragrant Heavens, Valerie Ann Worwood (Novato, California: New World Library, 1999).

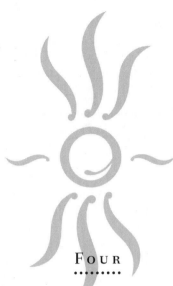

The Basic Techniques
of Subtle Energy Therapy

*O*ver the years, many techniques have been developed and utilized in subtle energy therapy that assist its unique ability to promote positive change and transformation. Intention, visualization, compassionate touch, and color are particularly valuable, and can be used alone or in combination with each other.

Intention and Visualization

The definitive foundation of subtle energy therapy is the intention to help another person. In the context of this book, intention is knowing and being clear about the purpose of the subtle energy session you give using compassionate touch. It is based on the premise that energy follows thought. Thinking about something is the first step to its manifestation, and there is nothing that has ever been accomplished that was not, at first, a thought. For this reason, your intention in giving a subtle energy session needs to reflect the purpose of the session in a positive and restorative way. The initial intention sets the stage to start, but intention is used throughout the session to direct the healing energy itself. An intention statement, or prayer, said aloud or silently, can be incorporated such as, "Let there be healing." A favorite of the authors is, "May this person be healed. May they receive what they need, and may all they receive be for their highest good and the highest good of all."

Visualization can also be used, and is another example of how energy follows thought. Shakti Gawain, in her classic book, *Creative Visualization*, says, "Simply having an idea or thought, holding it in your mind, is an energy which will tend to attract and create that form on the material plane." For example, it could be an image in your mind that a stiff knee is flexing comfortably, or that clogged nasal passages are draining and clearing to relieve a sinus headache.

Our hands are often the tools we use to manifest our intentions or visualizations in subtle energy therapy. Beautifully describing hands and their wondrous ability to help another person, Deborah Cowens says, "The hands are themselves great works of art. They possess beauty, power, and utility. In the hands, raw strength, miraculous precision, and musical dexterity become one. The hands can build bridges, sculpt stone, type, tie flies, and perform surgery. All the power of our minds, hearts, and souls are concentrated in our hands, which is why they are capable of re-shaping the world. Who can deny that they possess a unique and even awesome power? That power flows from your hands, and you can use it to heal."

A lovely poem by Dianne Neu, "Blessed Be the Work of Your Hands" found in *Earth Prayers From Around the World,* describes a spiritual dimension of using our hands, and how through them, each one of us has the ability to represent the Divine. It is interesting to note, in this spiritual context, that the philosopher Rudolph Steiner believed the human being can never become conscious of the Divine without touch.

Blessed be the work of your hands, O Holy One
Blessed be the hands that have touched life
Blessed be the hands that have nurtured and created
Blessed be the hands that have held pain
Blessed be the hands that have embraced with passion
Blessed be the hands that have tended gardens
Blessed be the hands that have closed in anger
Blessed be the hands that have planted new seeds
Blessed be the hands that have harvested ripe fields
Blessed be the hands that have cleaned, washed, mopped, and scrubbed
Blessed be the hands that have become knotty with age
Blessed be the hands that have wrinkled and scarred from doing justice
Blessed be the hands that have reached out and been received
Blessed be the hands that have held the promise of the future
Blessed be the works of your hands, O Holy One

78

Preparing Yourself and Your Hands

Though we all have the innate ability to heal with our hands, it is helpful to prepare yourself. To offer a subtle energy session with the intent to help someone else, the giver should be in a frame of mind that is as positive, relaxed, focused, and as supportive as possible. Each of these mental states contributes to the healing nature of a session. The hands must also be readied—engaged to send and direct the healing energy which flows directly out of the centers of the palms as well as the fingers. The following exercises will help you feel the energy more clearly, and help increase the strength of the energy.

Center in Your Breath

This exercise releases negative thoughts, and promotes focus and relaxation. Practice it as often as you can. Once familiar, you will quickly move through the steps, to accomplish the best attitude before giving a session.

Sit in a comfortable position.

Relax your eyes, letting them rest gently, half closed.

Take five deep breaths, and begin to notice the way your breath moves in and out of your body.

Notice the parts of your body that move with breathing, and the order in which they move. Notice how far the breath moves into your chest and belly, how much air you draw in, and how much you breathe out.

Give yourself the suggestion, "As I breathe out, I release all that is unbalanced on a physical, emotional, and spiritual level, that is ready to be released, and as I breath in, I am drawing in all the energy, and (add what is appropriate for you), that I need.

Now bring your awareness into your belly, and let any thoughts float in and out, observing them as if you were watching clouds float by in a big, blue sky.

Bring awareness to your breath again, and imagine how each cell in your body is being nourished and energized by it. Notice any thoughts, and come back to your breath.

Let the experience of centering in your breath bring you serenity, clarity, energy, and awareness.

Preparing Your Hands

Practice this three-part exercise as often as you can, and use it before you give a session. It takes only a few moments to complete. Put essential oil of lavender on your hands to strengthen the healing energy. Lavender also helps to increase your awareness of energy and your ability to feel it.

APPRECIATE YOUR HANDS.

Get into a comfortable sitting or standing position.

Take a few deep breaths to focus and energize.

Bring your awareness to your hands. Feel them and appreciate them.

Take a moment to reflect upon all the things your hands do everyday. Feel gratitude for them. They are remarkable!

Clear your mind and, again, focus on your hands. Feel and be aware of the differences of each part—the palm, the back, each finger, each knuckle, and each fingernail.

ACTIVATE YOUR HANDS.

Imagine, as you breathe, that you are sending breath directly into your hands. Notice how they may tingle, or change temperature.

Imagine that with your breath, you are activating your hands-turning on their energy receptors and preparing them to send healing energy.

Take a few moments to feel and experience this sensation.

GATHER AND PREPARE ENERGY FOR YOUR HANDS.

Bring your awareness into your first energy center (Base). Imagine that it is opening, drawing up earth energy as it grounds and replenishes. Let this earth energy move up through your energy centers to the fourth center (Heart).

Imagine your seventh center (Crown) opening, and a beautiful wave of pale, violet light pours into you, filling your Heart center, and bringing in spiritual strength, purpose, and guidance.

Allow both energies (earth and heaven) to co-mingle with the compassion of your Heart center. In this way, you are tapping into the infinite, bountiful resources of the universe. It is in your best interest to use this energy instead of your own to prevent depletion both energetically and emotionally.

Raise all these energies up into your fifth energy center (Throat), and allow them to pour down your shoulders and arms into your hands. Instruct this energy to keep flowing into and through you until the end of the session. Note: Many teachers suggest that healing energy be brought into the heart center (as in step C) to infuse it with love and move it out through the Throat center (as in this step) to connect it with Divine will.

The Role of Intuition

Practicing subtle energy therapy will help promote the opening and unfolding of intuition because they are both from the subtle realm. Intuition is the ability to perceive in a capacity that seems unrelated to the five other senses (seeing, touching, tasting, smelling, and hearing). Psychologist Frances Vaughan, in the transpersonal book, *The Inward Arc,* says that "intuition [is] a way of knowing that which transcends empirical and rational modes of knowing . . . given attention, it unfolds spontaneously."

Everyone has the capability to be intuitive. It is a creative capacity of the mind and tends to operate with insightful hunches such as "I don't know why, but I just had a feeling . . . .." Intuition becomes stronger the more you use and trust the process. It is not unusual for people giving subtle energy sessions to have strong feelings about changing a technique or even creating a new one. Pay attention to your intuition, and feel free to respond to it. Please note, however, that though intuition is remarkable and useful, like all human faculties, it is not one hundred percent infallible. Be certain to ask the receiver for feedback on all your techniques, including those that are based on intuition.

Using Color

Colors have a unique, vibrational and energetic signature that produces a specific effect in subtle energy therapy. There are seven colors in the visible light spectrum: red, orange, yellow, green, blue, indigo, and violet. These correlate to the seven primary energy centers. Visualizing and sending the appropriate color, combined with subtle energy techniques is optional, but can be helpful in bringing balance and harmony. Following is a chart of the color and energy center associations.

ENERGY CENTER	COLOR	EFFECTS
Base (1st)	Clear Red	Warming, revitalizing. Power, strength, courage.
Sacral (2nd)	Clear Orange	Warming, rejuvenating. Enthusiasm, optimism.
Solar Plexus (3rd)	Clear Yellow	Warming, inspiring. Knowledge, cheerfulness.
Heart (4th)	Clear Green	Balancing, relaxing, cleansing. Harmony, stability.
Throat (5th)	Clear Sky Blue	Cooling, calming. Concentration, introspection.
Third Eye (6th)	Clear Indigo Blue	Cooling, calming. Devotion, present awareness.
Crown (7th)	Clear Violet	Cooling, relaxing, restoring. Creativity, spirituality.

83

In addition to the energy centers, colors can be visualized on parts of the body to achieve a particular result. The soothing, vibrational qualities of blue can calm an inflamed condition, such as a sprained ankle. Red energizes, and can help in an area that has poor circulation, such as cold feet. Orange can bring joy to the heart, relieving emotional depression. Yellow can promote mental clarity, relieving confusion or worry when used around the head. Violet provides a protective boundary in a stressful situation when used to fill the auric field.

It addition to the seven prismatic colors, other colors can be useful such as pink and rose to promote love and compassion. White and gold are both related to high, spiritual vibrations, and are often used in meditations to contact the higher self and invoke the most sacred states of consciousness. Feel free to experiment with color and ask your receiver for feedback.

Some Terminology

In understanding techniques, here are some commonly used terms which may require explanations.

Balancing is the process of directing an energy center to achieve its optimal functioning—not too closed and not too expanded. When in a balanced state, a person can remain calm and centered in any situation. When out-of-balance, people tend to withdraw, be overwhelmed, or lose control of their emotions.

Grounded refers to a healthy, strong first (Base) energy center. For example, when we are well grounded, we are in the present, aware of our body, fully in our body, and well-connected to Mother Earth. We feel safe and secure in our earthly experience and love of life. People who are momentarily or chronically ungrounded may appear or feel confused and forgetful. They may experience great fear and a lack of trust in themselves, others, and the world at large. These people may be the dreamers who can't get anything done, or the spiritual ones who neglect to take care of their physical needs and day-to-day responsibilities.

Givers and receivers should both be properly grounded before a session begins so they are relaxed and aware at the same time. This is important for three reasons. 1) When grounded, the connection with earth provides us with energy that supports and revitalizes the Base energy center, our foundation. By doing this, all the bodies (subtle and physical) are linked, present, and grounded in the physical, and are more able to send and receive subtle energy. 2) Many of us are disassociated from our bodies and experiences. Rather than being in the present, we are thinking about the past or the future. Being grounded encourages us to be in the moment to experience a deeply therapeutic, in-the-body experience. 3) In order to provide the giver effective feedback, the receiver also needs to be aware of her body and what is being experienced. For example, if her back hurts, she may want a pillow under her knees. Once a person has been grounded, part of consciousness continues to be aware of the body, even in deep relaxation.

84

Linking energy centers refers to the process of connecting certain centers together in a particular way. Both essential oils and subtle energy techniques facilitate this process. Although the energy centers are always energetically linked and working together, there are times when we want to highlight the relationship and interdependence of two or more centers. For example, if we want to help someone to think more clearly when they feel in danger, our intention is focused on the partnership between the first center (feeling safe) and the sixth (thinking clearly). Linking lets us make these types of connections between the purpose and issues of the centers. In the following descriptions of hand placements, certain essential oils facilitate the connecting of certain energy centers. For example, sandalwood connects the first, second, and seventh energy centers, helping the different purposes and concerns of each center to become balanced and integrated. In this case, trust, sexuality, and spirit all support each other.

Connecting with an energy center refers to the process of the giver sending energy and intention into an energy center, and making contact so the center can become attuned to the giver. It is similar to tuning forks vibrating together. If they are in close proximity to each other, they will vibrate at the same frequency even if they had previously been vibrating at different frequencies when further apart. In subtle energy therapy, this connection can go both ways—the energy center begins to attune to the giver and the intention, and the giver begins to attune energetically to the needs of the energy center and receiver.

Healthy boundaries means the energy centers of the body are being opened and closed appropriately in any given situation. The boundary, which energetically is the actual outer boundary of the auric field, allows in that which nourishes us, and keeps out that which would harm us. In daily life, healthy boundaries help us prioritize, ask for what we need, and protect us from being depleted.

The 12 Basic Hand Positions for Subtle Energy Sessions

Gentle, compassionate touch, anywhere on the body, can be of great assistance to a person who is experiencing discomfort. Sometimes, this is all that is needed. Yet there are specific places and methods that the authors find particularly helpful. The following basic hand positions are simple yet powerful. Combined with corresponding essential oils, they form a foundation from which to begin your work with subtle energy. The essential oils are intended to be used singularly. However, in time and with experience, you may choose to blend them. Several essential oils are suggested for each position. Choose the one that is most appropriate for your receiver at the time.

After each position described below, we have included a visualization and color exercise that will assist you in keeping your intention clear and focused. They are not necessary but many givers find them to be helpful. An icon (✻) will mark these exercises.

The suggested time to hold each position is only a guideline, and with experience you will know when more or less time is appropriate. Remember, a drop of lavender rubbed on your palms will help you to develop this sensitivity. Preparation of the space or room in which a subtle energy session is given, and the preparation of the receiver is described in detail in Chapter 7. The section below is intended to teach the hand positions as they are used in a session, and are not a session by themselves.

Open Toes/Close Toes

Some practitioners have found that the tips of the toes correspond to the seven primary energy centers. Because there are five toes and seven energy centers, the connection is not one-to-one. The big toe connects with the first energy center, the baby toe connects with the sixth and seventh, and the other three toes work together on the remaining energy centers (second, third, fourth, and fifth). The most important consideration in this two-part technique is to be aware that touching the tips of each toe, from the biggest down to the smallest, grounds the receiver and opens the energy centers to receive healing energy at the beginning of a session.

Touching the baby toe up to the big toe gently closes the energy centers to the degree of openness that is best suited for daily living, at the end of a session.

The energy centers respond to our life experiences by opening or closing a bit, according to our awareness, intention, and need. In a healthy person, they remain somewhat open. In an emotionally or physically harmful situation, they partially close in order to protect us. When meditating or healing, they open to accept the positive influences.

Open Toes/Close Toes is based on Polarity therapy and is particularly important because most of us have imbalances in our energy centers. Some are more opened or closed than others, and there are times when our energy centers do not open and close appropriately. Because of trauma, misunderstanding, or confusion, harmful situations may not be recognized, and thus the energy centers do not respond to protect as they should. In other cases, healing energy may be unfamiliar and the energy centers won't open to receive it, or more commonly, only the upper centers open. In these

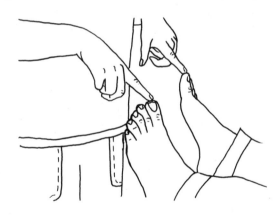

situations, we can use a combination of essential oils, energy, and intention to open and close each energy center when it is appropriate, creating healthy boundaries and grounded protection for our daily lives. A healthy boundary is not too rigid or too porous, but is like a semi-permeable cell membrane that lets in nourishment, and keeps out harm. Remember: if you open the energy centers, you must close them, appropriately.

Open Toes to begin each session. Using the tips of your index fingers, rest them on the tops of your receiver's big toes. Hold for five to ten seconds. Then move your index fingers, simultaneously and sequentially, to the tops of the second, third, fourth, and fifth toes.

✳ Visualize the opening of each energy center, consecutively, from the first to the seventh as if they were beautiful flowers or the wings of a butterfly. Visualize them in the colors of white, gold, or green.

Close Toes to end each session. Place your index fingers on the tops of the fifth toes and hold for five to ten seconds. Then touch and hold in succession the fourth, third, and second toes. Lastly, touch the big toes for ten seconds and then hold them, on top and bottom, between your thumbs and index fingers as you send the intention that the energy received by your receiver was for their highest good and the highest good of all.

✳ Visualize the energy centers as flowers closing to a bud or butterfly's wings folding against their body. Continue to visualize them in white, gold, or green.

Aromatherapy for Open/Close Toes

Vetiver grounds and balances all the energy centers. It also is protective as it assists in creating a safe place for energy sessions.

Lavender balances all the energy centers to the level of openness or closure best suited for the session.

Palmarosa sets the intention for healing, and supports the energy centers to allow what is needed.

Elemi used in Open Toes is grounding, and promotes deep relaxation and lucidity. Used in Close Toes, it brings back everyday reality, even after prolonged or deep relaxation.

Chamomile deeply relaxes and assists in opening to receive healing energy.

Head Hold

This is a technique that relaxes, balances, and relieves stress. Healing energy moves into the head and travels down the spine. This is a very helpful technique for anyone who is feeling agitated or ungrounded, and it can also help relieve neck or back pain. It is deeply comforting.

With the receiver reclining, gently lift the head, and rest it in your cupped palms. Form a cradle to support the back of the head. Find a position that is comfortable for your receiver, and then hold for three to five minutes.

Note: Do not overarch the neck. It should be comfortably positioned as if it were resting on a neck pillow. If your receiver has a neck or spine injury, place your hands lightly against the sides of their head, either touching or spacing your hands two to three inches away from the body.

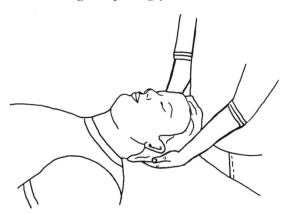

Send energy and hold for the same amount of time.

✳ Visualize an image that is tender and restful for you, like holding a sleeping baby or young animal in the palms of your hands. Send a gentle pink or rose color, filling the receiver with the vibration of compassion and love.

89

Aromatherapy for Head Hold

Lavender balances and connects each energy center as the subtle energy from this hold moves down the spine.

Sandalwood quiets the conscious mind, and encourages states of body/mind healing and meditation. It connects the first and the seventh energy centers, and supports all others by that connection.

Rosewood promotes a mental state comparable to meditation, allowing healing energy to be better received.

Frankincense deepens the breath and induces a meditative state. It helps to release the past, and prepare for healing in the present. It connects the 1st and 7th energy centers.

Cedarwood cuts through energy blocks and worry, and makes immediate contact with Divine energies.

Elemi balances the brain, promoting deep peace and profound lucidity. It unifies and balances the energy centers.

Forehead Spread

This is a Polarity therapy technique. It connects the sixth and seventh energy centers, and clears the mind so healing energy can be received. It is helpful for aches or uncomfortable symptoms in the head such as headaches, sinus congestion, eye strain, or neck tension. Do not use for migraines or migraines in progress.

Place both thumbs together, side by side, about two inches back from the hairline. Reach your index fingers towards the sixth energy center (Third Eye), as far as it is comfortable. Let your other fingers rest into a naturally-spaced spread across the forehead, holding firmly but gently with symmetrical, even pressure. Hold for one to three minutes.

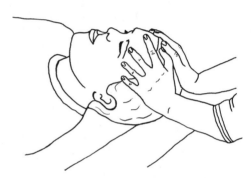

✳ Visualize sending a calming, deep indigo blue into the sixth energy center, and a lavender or white towards the seventh.

90

Aromatherapy for Forehead Spread

Rosemary works with the sixth energy center to integrate clarity and clairvoyance. It also provides psychic protection.

Rosewood opens the seventh center in preparation for subtle energy sessions. It modulates the opening so the receiver is not flooded with spiritual energies for which they are not prepared.

Sandalwood promotes a deeply receptive, meditative state of mind.

Lavender encourages deep stages of relaxation. It has a balancing effect, either energizing or relaxing, depending upon what is needed.

Elemi clears and relaxes the mind, and opens it to grounded, mystical experiences.

Cedarwood creates a direct link, through the seventh center, to Divine energies. It helps to promote the intention that the session will be for the highest good of the receiver, and for the highest good of all.

Angelica grounds the mind and body while opening them to the higher self and angelic energies.

Immortelle activates the intuitive and creative mind.

Combing and Smoothing the Auric Field

These are both common, popular energy-healing techniques from a variety of modalities. They are used to balance the auric field at the end of a session, help to replenish the field's boundaries, and to help remove debris that has been released during a session.

Combing. Hold your hands three to twelve inches away, directing your fingertips towards the receiver's body. Imagine light coming from each of your fingertips as if they were teeth in a comb. Begin at the head and move down one side and then the other, using long, combing, sweeping strokes. At the feet, sweep out and beyond the body, then shake your hands to release any debris that has been collected into the earth.

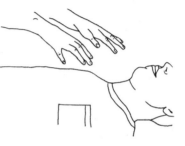

91

Smoothing. Slightly cup your hands. Using the same sweeping movements described above, smooth the auric field. Your hands may be further away from the body than for combing.

Remember to periodically shake your hands towards the ground to release energetic debris that has been collected.

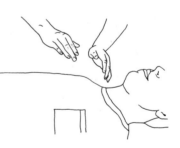

✳ While combing, visualize streams of white, pink, or gold light coming from each finger. While smoothing, fill your cupped palm with white, pink, or gold light. If you prefer, you can send a color that coordinates with the oils used such as rose for rose oil, lavender for lavender oil, yellow-orange for palmarosa, or a burnished gold for vetiver.

Aromatherapy for Combing and Smoothing the Auric Field

Rose gently fills holes in the auric field and seals it. It also grounds the
energy centers.

Lavender smooths and balances the auric field and the energy centers.
When used at the end of a subtle energy session, it helps to complete
the letting go of any released emotions or experiences in either the
physical or subtle bodies.

Palmarosa has a gentle nature that supports the healing energy experienced during and after a subtle energy session.

Vetiver balances, grounds, and helps to seal the auric field.

Filling

This is a gently energizing technique, well-suited for public places when
reclining is not possible or appropriate.

92

Place your palms on the shoulders or feet of the receiver. Feel the
earth's energy being drawn in through the bottom of your feet and filling
your fourth energy center (Heart). Visualize it moving to your fifth energy
center (Throat), down your arms, and then out your
hands to fill the receiver. Hold for five minutes.

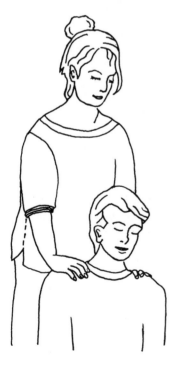

✳ Visualize a soft red, medium orange, or
sun yellow, pouring out of your hands and filling
the body from feet up or shoulders down until the
entire body is full of this colorful energy. Then visualize it overflowing out of the top of the head, or
out the bottoms of the feet, filling the auric field.

Aromatherapy for Filling

Lavender gently energizes.

Orange fills with joy.

Pine increases energy in all the subtle bodies.

Tangerine relieves feelings of emotional emptiness.

Frankincense and *rosemary* relieve mental fatigue.

Clary sage, geranium, and *rosemary* help to relieve
physical fatigue.

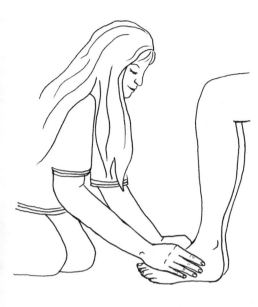

Simple Hold

Place your hands on either side of the area that needs attention—side to side or front to back. This technique can be done with your hands touching the body, or off the body in the auric field. Send a gentle wave from one hand to the other until the energy flow feels even or continuous, or until you sense that it is finished. If you are using one hand or one hand on top of the other, gently send energy until you sense the area is full.

Note: As you practice, you will discover your own way of knowing when the hold is finished. Some people see an image of completion, others sense a tingling in their hands, and others just know. There is no right or wrong way. In the beginning, you may feel more comfortable holding for a prescribed amount of time—we recommend three to five minutes.

93

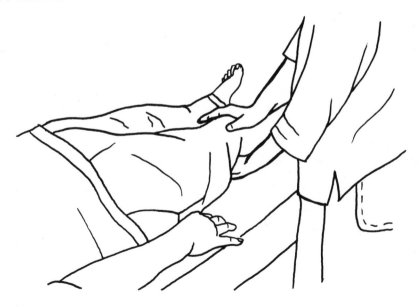

The following hand placements for Simple Hold are based on Reiki guidelines. They are very helpful for specific situations.

Hands cupped over the eyes	Relieves anxiety, reduces stress, relaxes, and promotes mental clarity.
Hands covering the temples	Relieves worry, reduces stress, and promotes calmness and mental clarity.
Hands over the back of the head	Reduces fear and worry, relieves stress, and promotes a sense of well-being.
Hands over the throat	Relieves anger, resentment, and frustration, and promotes feelings of security.
Hands over the heart	Promotes relaxation and reduces stress.
Hands over the liver/stomach	Reduces stress and anxiety, relieves frustration, and promotes self-confidence.
Hands over the lower belly	Releases anger and fear, and promotes greater creativity.
Hands cupping over the ears	Promotes receptivity to inner and outer information.
Hands on the ankles	Releases tension and stress.
Hands on the knees	Releases tension and stress, releases emotions, and promotes forgiveness.
Hands on the wrists	Releases tension and stress, and promotes creative expression.
Hands on elbows	Releases tension and stress, and promotes interaction with the environment.
Hands on the shoulders	Releases tension and stress, and motivates.

94

✱ Visualize an appropriate color (such as blue for inflammation, or pink for love), moving back and forth between your hands, glowing clear and bright and strong.

Aromatherapy for Simple Hold

In this position, essential oils can be chosen and used to address four different issues.

1) Physical. Use the oils that assist with the physical condition. For example, use eucalyptus for a cold over the lungs, peppermint for indigestion over the stomach, or rosemary over the location of muscle aches.

2) Energy centers. Different organs and body parts are related to the various energy centers (see Chapter 1). Choose an oil appropriate for the energy center or the affected part. For example, for congestion in the lungs use oils good for the fourth energy center such as rose or bergamot. For a headache, use oils good for the sixth or seventh energy center such as lemon or sandalwood.

3) Mental/Emotional issues. Hold the energy center related to the issue (see Chapter 1 as a reference), or the place on the body where the receiver feels the symptom. For example, fear is often felt in the neck and shoulders, chest, or belly. Use the oils that address the issue. Orange alleviates depression and brings feelings of joy; cedarwood calms down a worried mind; ylang ylang relaxes to reduce fear; rosemary reduces mental confusion; sandalwood increases self-esteem; marjoram assists with grief; chamomile reduces irritability.

4) Subtle energy. Use for the energy centers and subtle bodies. Choose an oil that meets the appropriate need such as benzoin to energize and fill a depleted area; black pepper to remove energy blocks; juniper to cleanse, clear congestion, and help energy flow; lavender to balance, release stagnated energy if congested and bring energy to the area if depleted; lemon to cleanse energetically; palmarosa to use as a general tonic that supports energy; rosemary to help energy to move and flow; and pine to amplify energy while it removes negative energy or blocks and strengthens energy flow.

Brain Balance

The two hemispheres of the brain are related to two different types of mental processes or thinking, though this is not a rigid correlation. The right brain is used during tasks that are creative or intuitive. The left brain is used primarily during tasks that require rational processing. In order to have a powerful, creative, clear, insightful mind, both capacities need to be available and work together equally. The brain balance technique can help with symptoms of an unbalanced right and left brain condition such as confusion, headache, worry, over-thinking, and creative blocks.

Place your palms against the sides of your receiver's head, in a position comfortable for both of you. Gently send a wave of energy from the palm of your left hand through the head to your right hand. When you feel the right hand receive the energy, gently send it back to the left. Interestingly, it will usually take longer for the wave to move in one direction than the other. The goal of this technique is to continue until the energy is moving back and forth at an equal rate. It may be fast or slow, but it should be balanced. This usually takes about five minutes but can take much longer if someone is in physical or mental distress.

Note: Ask your receiver if they suffer from dizziness or motion sickness. If they do, you may need to avoid this technique as it might upset their stomach.

96

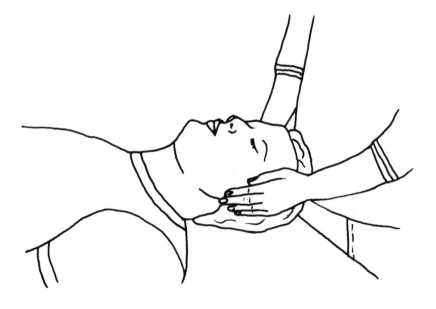

✻   Imagine a slender ray of lavender light moving from one hand to the other. Then imagine that the lavender begins to increase in size, gradually filling the entire head and radiating out into the auric field.

Aromatherapy for Brain Balance

Rosemary connects with, balances, and clarifies the logical mind (left brain).

Immortelle opens the intuitive mind (right brain) and is helpful for any type of creative blocks.

Lavender relaxes, clarifies, and balances.

Pine energizes and relieves feelings of mental sluggishness.

Jasmine balances, and is good when the mind is in conflict, especially when trying to make a decision.

Cedarwood releases worry and mental blocks. It opens the seventh center to Divine energy throughout the physical and subtle bodies.

Thyme activates and supports the left brain without causing an imbalance with the right brain.

Energy Ball

This is an earth-energy healing technique that re-energizes the body, and is especially good when your receiver is feeling depleted from stress or illness, or is soon to face a stressful situation. It is more intensely energizing than the Filling technique.

Vigorously rub your hands together. Then gently pump your hands together and apart to build up energy until it is about the size of a soccer ball. (See the exercises in Chapter 1.) Hold the energy ball above your receiver's midsection, and slowly release the ball while gently directing it into his/her body. Your hands will then be resting on the stomach area. Notice whether the receiver's body wants to receive all the energy. If you feel a resistance, it means your receiver has enough. Do not force it, as it may cause nausea.

Note: If your receiver has suffered a recent psychological attack, such as being the brunt of someone's rage, complete this technique by moving your right hand counterclockwise over the third energy center to seal and protect.

✳ Imagine a shining ball of yellow, orange, or red light building between your hands. Now imagine that as it moves into the receiver's midsection, their whole torso, front and back, begins to glow with that light.

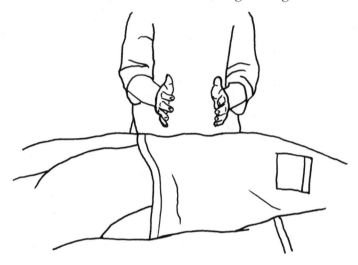

98

Aromatherapy for Energy Ball

Choose the oil based upon the original cause of energy depletion.

Orange energizes with feelings of joy and so helps with depression or listlessness.

Benzoin energizes and is especially good to dispel depletion caused by worry or other mental over use.

Black pepper is a mental stimulant and is useful when the receiver is feeling frustrated from being stuck.

Pine increases energy in the body while it repels negativity. It connects with and balances the physical and etheric bodies.

Juniper, rosemary, and *fennel* all energize as well as clear the body of any effects of negativity. They also help to seal and protect.

Melissa is helpful when depletion is caused by grief.

Windshield Wipers

This is a Polarity therapy technique that is designed to gently massage and balance the physical and subtle bodies. With the receiver lying on their

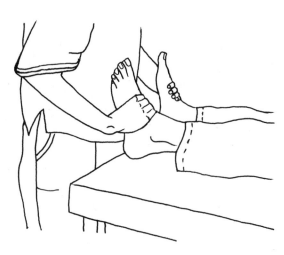

back, stand at the feet. Gently lift your receiver's feet and move the legs outwards to the edge of the table. With your hands holding the feet on the tops or at the sides, begin a slow, gentle, rhythmic, parallel rocking movement—both feet to the right, then both to the left, as windshield wipers. Slowly stop and hold the feet quietly for a moment. Alternate and repeat this rocking and holding two more times.

 Visualize the energy centers in the bottom of your feet drawing in the earth's energy in a deep, clear, warm golden color, and sending it to your receiver.

Aromatherapy for Windshield Wipers

Lavender helps to balance all the energy centers.

Sandalwood connects the first and seventh energy centers, and is relaxing.

Vetiver grounds, balances, and protects the centers.

Patchouli helps to re-attach and ground when a person is disoriented.

Myrrh grounds and nourishes the first center, and helps to release feelings of being stuck by promoting flexibility and movement.

Oakmoss is grounding and strengthening especially during spiritual, meditative, or energy work.

Pine releases negative energy while increasing positive energy throughout the spine and energy centers.

Orange gently energizes and provides support.

Grounding Wave

This is an earth-energy healing technique that is useful for people who are ungrounded. It is helpful for people who feel as if they are in a daze, or are experiencing confusion.

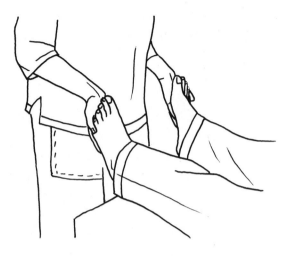

Place your hands on the bottoms of your receiver's feet in a comfortable position. Begin to send waves of energy up through the center of your receiver's body following the spine. Allow the waves to set their own pace—fast or slow, long or short. As the waves move out the top of the head, let them reach out to catch any energy that extends inappropriately out of the top of the head. Now begin to reverse the wave and bring it back down—into the receiver's feet and into your hands. You will sense when all the receiver's energy is back in their body. Some people see it, some feel a "click", and some feel the feet getting warmer. Remember to disconnect slowly.

✳ Visualize a wave of deep, bright red light waving through the body. When the wave returns and is completed, imagine each energy center alive and alight with its own beautiful color.

Aromatherapy for Grounding Wave

Elemi helps bring the receiver back to ordinary reality after deep meditation.
Oakmoss is grounding during energy work and spiritual practices.
Patchouli strengthens and grounds. It helps re-attach the spirit to the
    physical body when the spirit has moved out during spiritual work,
    healing, or trauma.
Vetiver grounds, balances all energy centers and protects the auric field.
Ylang ylang and *tea tree* help recovery from shock.

Cleansing Spin

This technique is based on material from Alice Bailey's Esoteric Healing. It is a powerful way to clear the auric field of any thought-forms or feelings that have been released from one level of the auric field during the session, but may be trapped in another level. It creates an energy vortex that lifts debris out and away from your receiver and sends it into the earth.

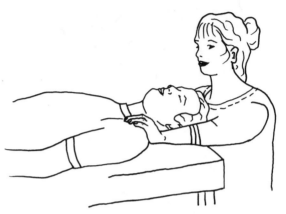

Sit or stand at the head or to the side of your receiver, and gently rest your hands on their body. Place your awareness just beyond their auric field above their head, usually a couple of feet away. Now imagine a wide, swirling white energy whirling around the receiver, clockwise. Allow the vortex to move all the way down the body, spinning two to three feet into the earth, where it dissipates. Keep the vortex spinning for three to five minutes, until you sense that the auric field is cleared.

101

At the completion of the cleansing, visualize the receiver's auric field to be a clear, shining, white light shaped like a large egg and totally surrounding the entire body.

Aromatherapy for Cleansing Spin

Juniper cleanses and detoxifies the physical and subtle bodies. It clears negative energies and negative self-concepts.

Lavender releases emotional patterns and helps clear the astral body.

Vetiver cleanses all levels of the auric field and provides protection.

Eucalyptus clears negativity and is excellent after releasing anger.

Rosemary releases negativity and outmoded thought forms from the mental body.

Energy Center Balancing

This is a Polarity therapy technique from Becky Williams at Twin Lakes College of the Healing Arts. It is used to balance all the energy centers. It is the most complicated of the techniques but is very rewarding to learn. The gentle rocking and holding is soothing and relaxing, and allows equilibrium to occur in a gentle way. This process helps to release any blockages in the energy centers, as well as distribute energy in the energy system pathway along the spine.

The receiver lies comfortably face down. Stand on their left side so your left hand can gently contact their neck—your thumb on one side, your fingers wrapped around the other side, or make contact with your hand in a cupped position. Your left hand will remain in this position throughout the exercise. Now, place your right hand at the first energy center, lengthwise along the spine, palm facing upwards, fingers pointing towards the head. Keep your hand there for thirty to sixty seconds. Then rotate your right hand so that it is resting across the spine, perpendicular, turning the palm downward. Gently rock the right hand for twenty to thirty seconds. Slowly come to a stop, and let the hand rest for thirty seconds.

Now move your right hand up to the second energy center, and place it in alignment with the spine, palm down. Hold for thirty to sixty seconds. Then rotate your right hand ninety degrees so it rests across or perpendicular to the spine (your hands are now parallel), and repeat the rocking process. Repeat for the third and fourth energy centers.

To end, raise your hands gently off the body.

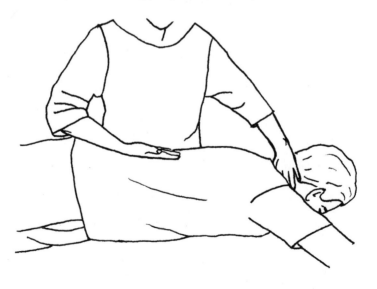

✳ Visualize a beautiful, soft, blue light moving out of your left hand into the neck, and with your right hand, send red into the first center, orange into the second, yellow into the third, and green into the fourth. Imagine each energy center being round and full as it draws in the energy and light.

Aromatherapy for Energy Center Balancing

For energy centers that need particular attention, choose an essential oil that is appropriate for that center.

Lavender balances all the energy centers.

Vetiver balances all the energy centers, grounds, and protects the auric field.

Pine increases energy in the auric field and protects it.

103

Recommended Reading

Subtle Aromatherapy, Patricia Davis (England: C. W. Daniels Co. Ltd., 1991).

Hands-on Healing, Jack Angelo (Rochester, VT: Healing Arts Press, 1994).

Empowerment through Reiki, Paula Horan (Twin Lakes, WI: Lotus Light Publications, 1990).

Accepting Your Power to Heal: The Personal Practice of Therapeutic Touch, Dolores Krieger, Ph.D. (Santa Fe, NM: Bear and Company Publications, 1993).

Your Hands Can Heal, Ric A. Weinman (New York: Penguin Books, 1992).

You Already Know What to Do, Sharon Franquemont (New York, Tarcher/ Putman, 1999).

FIVE

Using Essential Oils as Subtle Energy Therapy

*A*romatherapy and other techniques of subtle energy therapy stand alone in their ability to promote and support the well-being of body, mind, and spirit. However, using them together creates a new dimension, and reaps a synergistic reward. Essential oils, chosen for their appropriate energetic properties, gently yet profoundly amplify the capacity and effects of subtle energy healing techniques, especially compassionate touch.

Using Essential Oils with Intention

We have discussed intention as the basis of subtle energy therapy. Due to this, intention plays a role with using essential oils for energy healing. It is imperative to be clear about how you want the essential oils to help you. The capacity of purposeful thought to amplify the healing effects of a substance has been reported by Dr. Larry Dossey in his book, *Healing Words*. He describes experiments in which subtle energy therapists held bottles of water with the intention of sending healing energy into the water. "Samples of the water were added to solutions of yeast cells . . . statistically significant increases in carbon dioxide were observed in the yeast cultures given the 'treated' water."

In another series of experiments illustrating the effect of intention, Oskar Estibany, an energy healer, held a one percent saline solution which would usually retard the normal growth of barley seeds. The experiments discovered ". . . that the damaging effect of the saline could be inhibited if Estibany held the container of saline for fifteen minutes." We conclude that positive intention for healing can influence a substance. For our purposes, it intensifies the beneficial, subtle effects of essential oils.

Methods of Using Essential Oils

The primary methods of using essential oils in subtle energy therapy are diffusion, anointing, and sprays or mists. Giving subtle energy sessions offers many opportunities to employ each of these methods, working with the overall energetics and subtle bodies of the receiver, or the individual energy centers.

METHOD	RECIPE	PURPOSE	APPLICATION
Diffuser	Follow diffuser manufacturer's instructions.	To clear and cleanse a room. To bring in positive energy. To affect consciousness. To ask for guidance.	Used in a room or area.
As an anointing oil	Dilute essential oil(s) in a carrier oil, such as jojoba or olive. Use 5-10 drops of essential oil in one tablespoon of carrier oil. (The fragrance will be delicate. Remember, using essential oils in subtle energy therapy requires a low amount.	To set up boundaries. To ask for guidance. To use with subtle energy techniques.	To apply to the appropriate energy center with the fingertip. To stroke above the energy center or the auric field with the hands.
As a spray/mist	Add 10-15 drops to 4 oz. of spring water in a misting bottle.	To clear and cleanse a room. To bring in positive energy. To set up boundaries. To affect consciousness. To use with subtle energy techniques.	Mist a room, your hands, and/or the receiver. (Remember to place a sheet over the receiver so the oils won't stain clothes.)

Techniques for Using Essential Oils in Subtle Energy Therapy

The four fundamental purposes for using essential oils in a hands-on, subtle energy session are: setting sacred space, affecting consciousness, preparing yourself, and working with the receiver's energy centers. Some methods are better suited than others for each purpose. For example, anointing is the preferred method for preparing yourself. Misting is a good way to clear and cleanse the area, and a diffuser is well-suited for bringing in positive energy.

Setting Sacred Space

We believe that all forms of subtle energy therapy, as well as any type of healing, is sacred. To acknowledge this spiritual dimension, we suggest you dedicate the room or area in which the subtle energy session is given to that which is greater than ourselves—to God, guidance, spirit, or whatever is meaningful for you. There are four important steps to create a sacred space. However, if you do not have time to go through all of them, choose a multi-purpose oil such as lavender or cedarwood, and as you mist the room, intend that it accomplishes all of the following.

1) Clear and cleanse the area of past experiences, and ready it for a new experience by misting or diffusing essential oils. Choose one of the single oils or use the blend below.

Cedarwood and *juniper* are the primary oils used for this purpose.

Pine, lavender, rosemary, and *lemon* are also good as general cleansers.

Eucalyptus is good to clear the air after an argument or intense session where negative thoughts or feelings have been released.

Clearing and Cleansing Blend

5 drops cedarwood

3 drops lemon

2 drops eucalyptus

2) Bring in positive energy by misting or diffusing the area once again with one of the following oils or with the blend.

Bergamot and *orange* promote joy, cheerfulness, and optimism.
Cedarwood strengthens the connection with the Divine.
Lavender calms and balances.
Neroli instills comfort and strength.
Petitgrain promotes optimism.
Rose promotes love and compassion.
Rosewood promotes self acceptance.
Vetiver calms and grounds.

Positive Energy Blend

4 drops orange

3 drops lavender

3 drops rose

3) Set up energy boundaries to provide the giver protection from negative thoughts and feelings. Mist the room and/or the giver, or apply as an anointing oil. Choose one of the following single oils or use the blend.

Fennel protects against negative psychic influence.
Rosemary strengthens self-confidence and is a spiritual protector.
Juniper clears negativity and protects against other people's influence.
Lemon promotes trust and security.
Vetiver protects against over-sensitivity.

Boundary Blend

4 drops juniper

4 drops lemon

2 drops rosemary

110

4) Ask for guidance by diffusing or applying as an anointing oil. The giver places one drop on his or her sixth energy center (Third Eye).

Cedarwood and *neroli* connects us with our higher self.

Rose, jasmine, and *angelica* welcome the influence of angels.

Chamomile (both Roman and German), lavender, geranium, and *frankincense* bring in healing guides and help us to experience their presence.

Guidance Blend

5 drops jasmine

3 drops lavender

2 drops cedarwood

Affecting Consciousness

Use essential oils to create a state of mind for the highest good of the giver and receiver during a subtle energy session by diffusing or misting the room. Many essential oils can be used for this purpose. The following are a few examples:

Frankincense to slow and deepen the breath, creating a sense of calm,

Ylang ylang to promote feelings of peace, serenity, and joy,

Sandalwood to promote inner unity with mind, body, and spirit,

Bergamot to help heal a wounded heart,

Lemon to uplift and clarify the mind.

Preparing Yourself

After the environment has been cleansed and filled with positive energy, place a drop of a grounding, anointing oil on your feet, such as patchouli or vetiver. Next, anoint your hands with a drop of lavender. Rub them together to help activate the energy in your hands and make them more sensitive. A drop of rose on your heart brings compassion to the work of your hands.

Working with the Energy Centers

Much of a subtle energy session involves working with the individual energy centers with intent to bring them into balance. Imbalances in the energy centers may be due to too much energy (congestion), or too little energy (constriction). Essential oils and hands-on, subtle energy techniques restore harmony and balance to the energy centers by coming into contact with them and vibrating at the center's healthiest frequency. Many essential oils have an affinity with specific energy centers, supporting and promoting the healthy cellular vibrational patterns of that center. Employing the appropriate essential oil makes the subtle energy techniques more effective.

The following are directions for each method when using them during a session for a specific energy center. One or more techniques can be used during a single session.

Misting. Gently spray the area above the appropriate energy center.

Stroking. Put a drop of an anointing oil on your left palm, rub your hands together and stroke or rest your hand in the area where it is needed, without touching the body. Commonly, your hands will be three to six inches away from the body.

Anointing. Place a drop on your fingertip, and then touch the energy center where it is needed.

Additional Techniques. To help balance a particular energy center:

1) Allow the receiver to smell the appropriate essential oil on a tissue or cotton swab. Ask them to imagine drawing its fragrance into the energy center.

2) Place a drop of the appropriate anointing oil under your receiver's nose so they can experience its subtle fragrance, drawing the scent into the energy center.

3) Use the stroking technique combined with color. Imagine the color associated with the energy center radiating from your hands into the center.

Following is a list of the energy centers with their associated essential oils, common imbalances with suggested essential oils to restore equilibrium, and recipes for essential oil blends.

Note: Whenever possible, let the receiver smell the chosen essential oil or blend before using it to be certain that they like the fragrance. It will be difficult for them to have a positive experience if the scent is offensive. If someone has a negative reaction, choose another oil appropriate for the center, and let them smell it again until you find one they like.

First Energy Center-Root or Base
ESSENTIAL OILS

Benzoin Grounds and comforts.

Cedarwood Connects us with earthly forces.

Coriander Promotes feelings of security and earthly contentment.

Frankincense Calms and centers. Links base with the crown.

Marjoram Comforts and supports.

Myrrh Strengthens, energizes and supports.

Oakmoss Grounds. Increases sense of prosperity and security.

Patchouli Strengthens and grounds. Good for people who are over thinking.

Peru Balsam Promotes feelings of being safe and secure.

Sandalwood Promotes inner unity—re-aligning body, mind, and spirit. Grounds and connects us with our sense of being.

Vanilla Promotes feelings of safety and comfort.

Vetiver Balances, grounds, and protects. Promotes strength and a deep sense of belonging.

COMMON IMBALANCES

Constricted energy:

Difficulty in giving and taking—lemon, rosewood, frankincense.

Disconnected from body—patchouli, frankincense, rosewood.

Underweight—frankincense, jasmine.

Weak physical constitution—myrrh, frankincense.

Experiencing life on earth as a burden—frankincense, patchouli.

Fearful—ylang ylang, sandalwood.

Undisciplined—frankincense, rosemary.

Disorganized—vetiver, lavender, rosemary.

Congested energy:
  Materialistic—lemon, clary sage, juniper.
  Overweight—cypress, orange.
  Self-indulgent—lemon, orange, sandalwood.
  Ignores needs of others—lemon, orange, sandalwood.
  Sluggish—lemon, myrrh, lavender.
  Quick to anger, aggression—chamomile, ylang ylang, rosewood.
  Possessive—cypress, ylang ylang, lavender.

Base Energy Center Blends

For integrating body and spirit; remaining grounded during meditation:
  6 drops cedarwood
  2 drops sandalwood
  2 drops oakmoss
  1 T. jojoba oil

For increasing basic trust in the goodness of the universe:
  6 drops frankincense
  4 drops peru balsam
  1 T. jojoba oil

For balancing the mind and emotions while grounding the physical body:
  3 drops patchouli
  3 drops vanilla
  4 drops sandalwood
  1 T. jojoba oil

Second Energy Center-Sacral
ESSENTIAL OILS

Cardamom Stimulates sexual energy.

Coriander Increases creativity, spontaneity, and passion.

Geranium Nourishes feminine creativity, and promotes relaxed spontaneity.

Jasmine Connects spirituality and sexuality. Promotes creativity and artistic development.

Neroli Connects spirituality and sensuality. Promotes sensual comfort.

Orange Promotes joy in sexuality and creativity.

Patchouli Facilitates enjoyment of the senses and awakening of creativity.

Peru Balsam Promotes sensuality and confidence.

Rose Connects sexuality with the Heart center. Promotes creativity and love of beauty.

Sandalwood Connects sensuality with spirituality. Increases sexual energy.

Vanilla Increases feelings of sensuality.

Ylang Ylang Promotes sensuality. Helps unite our emotional and sexual natures.

COMMON IMBALANCES
Constricted energy:

Suppressed sexual desires—sandalwood, rose, jasmine.

Negative attitude about sexuality—patchouli, sandalwood, rose.

Nervous about sexuality—ylang ylang, sandalwood, jasmine.

Poor social skills—geranium, lemon, cypress, ylang ylang.

Unable to appreciate the miracle of life—orange, rose, sandalwood.

Lack of self-esteem—juniper, sandalwood, ylang ylang.

Lack of passion, excitement—jasmine, sandalwood, patchouli.

Frigidity—jasmine, rose, sandalwood.

Congested energy:

Sexual addiction—rose, clary sage.

Strong emotions, mood swings—lavender, eucalyptus, geranium, rosewood.

115

Too sensitive—lemon, sandalwood, ylang ylang.

Emotionally dependent—rose, jasmine, ylang ylang.

Obsessive attachment—clary sage, sandalwood, rose.

Sacral Energy Center Blends

For increasing sexual energy:

 6 drops cardamom

 4 drops vanilla

 1 T. jojoba oil

For supporting a safe, loving, sensual, and spiritual sexuality:

 5 drops rose

 5 drops sandalwood

 1 T. jojoba oil

For promoting sensual joy:

 6 drops orange

 3 drops sandalwood

 1 drop ylang ylang

 1 T. jojoba oil

Third Energy Center-Solar Plexus
Essential Oils

Cedarwood Strengthens confidence and will.

Chamomile, Roman Encourages calm acceptance of our own limitations.

Ginger Promotes courage and confidence.

Juniper Protects against negative influences. Restores confidence.

Peppermint Helps to overcome feelings of inferiority.

Petitgrain Promotes a healthy self-esteem.

Pine Restores self-confidence and strength of will.

Rosemary Protects from external influences. Boosts self-confidence. Promotes action.

Rosewood Promotes self-acceptance.

Tea Tree Builds confidence.

Thyme Promotes self-confidence.

Vetiver Protects against over-sensitivity.

Common Imbalances

Constricted energy:

Low energy—juniper, rosemary, lemon, lavender.

Inner discontent—lemon, tangerine, ylang ylang, rosewood.

Low self-esteem—juniper, sandalwood, ylang ylang, rosemary, petitgrain.

Weak willed—cypress, vetiver.

Easily upset—peppermint, juniper, fennel.

Easily discouraged—lemon, orange, tangerine.

Inhibited emotional expression—marjoram, ylang ylang, sandalwood.

Conforms for acceptance—frankincense, petitgrain, peppermint.

Easily stressed in challenging situations—lavender, sandalwood, ylang ylang, frankincense.

Unreliable—frankincense, vetiver, sandalwood.

Congested energy:

Manipulative and controlling—rosewood, vetiver, peppermint.

Desire to be powerful—petitgrain, vetiver, lemon.

Unable to relax—lavender, juniper, tangerine, cedarwood.

117

Always needs to be right—vetiver, juniper, rosemary.
Temper outbursts—chamomile (either), vetiver, lavender, ylang ylang.
Stubborn—cypress, juniper, lemon.
Arrogant—petitgrain, rosemary, lemon.
Hyperactive—chamomile, lavender, geranium.

Solar Plexus Energy Center Blends

For increasing positive sense of self-esteem and confidence:

7 drops rosewood

3 drops ginger

1 T. jojoba oil

For releasing negative energy or clearing energy blockages:

7 drops juniper

3 drops rosemary

1 T. jojoba oil

For releasing negative messages from the past and promoting healthy self-esteem:

7 drops petitgrain

2 drops juniper

1 drop rosemary

1 T. jojoba oil

Fourth Energy Center-Heart

ESSENTIAL OILS

Bergamot Opens the heart and allows love to radiate. Especially good for grief.

Immortelle Promotes compassion for others and oneself.

Jasmine Warms and opens the heart. Promotes heartfelt expression.

Lavender Calms and stabilizes emotions of the heart.

Lemon Helps to open the heart, easing fears of emotional involvement.

Marjoram Helps us to accept deep, emotional loss. Promotes ability to give.

Mimosa Opens the heart to receive love.

Melissa Relieves emotional blocks from grief. Promotes understanding and acceptance.

Myrrh Eases sorrow and grief.

Palmarosa Comforts the heart. Relieves emotional clinging.

Rose Promotes love especially when the heart is wounded by grief. Harmonizes. Restores self-confidence and strength of will.

Rosemary Inspires faith and joyful love.

Spikenard Promotes hope. Comforts those who take on the suffering of the world.

Tuberose Expands our capacity to give and receive love.

Valerian Comforts the wounded heart.

Yarrow, blue Increases healthy love for ourself and others.

COMMON IMBALANCES

Constricted energy:

Anti-social—bergamot, melissa, jasmine.

Disappointed when love is not returned—jasmine, rose, melissa.

Unable to receive love—bergamot, jasmine, rosewood.

Intolerant of others—eucalyptus, chamomile (either), ylang ylang.

Fear of intimacy—rose, jasmine, lavender, ylang ylang.

Overly sensitive—spikenard, lavender, sandalwood.

Dependent on love from others—bergamot, rose, spikenard.

Depressed—neroli, orange, sandalwood.

Cold and indifferent—jasmine, rose, sandalwood.

Congested energy:

Co-dependent—spikenard, bergamot, ylang ylang, cypress.

Demanding—black pepper, eucalyptus, rosewood.

Jealous—bergamot, rose, cypress, ylang ylang.

Over-attachment—spikenard, lavender, peppermint.

Gives too much of oneself—spikenard, bergamot, cypress.

Heart Energy Center Blends

For helping to heal a heart wounded by grief:

7 drops bergamot

3 drops rose

1 T. jojoba oil

For supporting the heart during times of painful change:

4 drops bergamot

4 drops melissa

2 drops yarrow

1 T. jojoba oil

For encouraging trust in the wisdom of the heart:

5 drops rose

4 drops jasmine

1 drop immortelle

1 T. jojoba oil

120

Fifth Energy Center-Throat
ESSENTIAL OILS
Chamomile, German Allows one to express truth calmly and without anger.
Chamomile, Roman Helps one to express spiritual truth.
Fennel Promotes uninhibited communication.
Geranium Increases capacity to listen, and communicate intimately.
Myrrh Supports one who is non-communicative due to lack of confidence.
Peppermint Promotes clarity in communication.

COMMON IMBALANCES
Constricted energy:
> Fear of speaking—German chamomile, cinnamon, myrrh
> Weak voice—German chamomile, myrrh
> Inability to express deep feelings or true self—German chamomile, geranium, rose, jasmine
> Shy or withdrawn—myrrh, ylang ylang, peppermint

Congested energy:
> Speaks harshly—German chamomile, geranium, ylang ylang
> Talks too much—German chamomile, cypress, lavender
> Inability to listen—geranium, chamomile, lavender

Throat Energy Center Blends
For developing effective communication skills that support the growth of intimacy in relationships:
> 5 drops German chamomile
> 5 drops geranium
> 1 T. jojoba oil

For identifying, understanding, and communicating one's deepest spiritual truth and knowledge:
> 5 drops Roman chamomile
> 5 drops myrrh
> 1 T. jojoba oil

121

For speaking our wisdom from a clear, grounded, protected place:
    6 drops geranium
    2 drops myrrh
    2 drops Roman chamomile
    1 T. jojoba oil

Sixth Energy Center-Third Eye or Brow
ESSENTIAL OILS

Basil Clears the mind.

Bay Laurel Promotes psychic awareness. Opens us to new thoughts and perspectives.

Cedarwood Clears and strengthens the mind.

Cinnamon leaf Increases psychic abilities.

Clary sage Strengthens the inner eye, helping us to see more clearly.

Clove Strengthens the conscious mind. Assists in recovering memories.

Fir Increases intuition.

Frankincense Quiets and clarifies the mind.

Grapefruit Increases intuition.

Immortelle Activates the intuitive right side of the brain.

Jasmine Opens the mind to visions of deeper truths. Enhances intuition and creative thinking.

Juniper Assists clairvoyance, but only if used for altruistic reasons. Dispels mental stagnation.

Lemon Uplifts and clarifies the mind.

Lemongrass Stimulates psychic awareness.

Neroli Reunites the conscious and subconscious.

Palmarosa Develops wisdom.

Peppermint Promotes inspiration and insights. Stimulates the conscious mind.

Petitgrain Stimulates the conscious mind and clears perception.

Rosemary Promotes clear thoughts, insights, and understanding.

Sandalwood Helps calm mental chatter.

Yarrow, blue Increases and focuses psychic awareness.

123

COMMON IMBALANCES

Constricted energy:

Insensitive—juniper, chamomile (either), lavender.

Out of touch with reality—rosemary, thyme.

No inner life—neroli, cedarwood, rose.

Poor memory—rosemary, thyme.

Forgetfulness—cedarwood, rosemary.

Confusion—cedarwood, rosemary, thyme.

Impaired vision—rosemary, rose, sandalwood.

Congested energy:

Too intellectual—immortelle, clary sage, lavender.

Intellectual arrogance—cedarwood, rosemary, lemon.

Rejects spirituality—juniper, neroli, Roman chamomile.

Difficulty concentrating—rosemary, cedarwood, eucalyptus.

Nightmares—rosemary, frankincense, lavender.

Third Eye Energy Center Blends

For developing mental clarity and objectivity:

5 drops lemon

3 drops basil

2 drops rosemary

1 T. jojoba oil

For supporting the development of inner vision and psychic abilities:

5 drops clary sage

3 drops lemon

2 drops sandalwood

1 T. jojoba oil

For releasing worry and fear so that we can receive and trust our intuitive guidance:

5 drops jasmine

3 drops neroli

2 drops grapefruit

1 T. jojoba oil

Seventh Energy Center-Crown
ESSENTIAL OILS

Angelica Connects us with angelic guidance. Aligns us with our higher selves.

Benzoin Steadies and focuses the mind for meditation or prayer.

Cedarwood Restores a sense of spiritual certainty. Strengthens connection with the Divine.

Elemi Balances spiritual practices with worldly responsibilities.

Frankincense Connects us with the eternal and Divine. Strengthens spiritual consciousness and aspirations.

Galbanum Connects us with Divine trust and innocence.

Hyssop Heightens spirituality.

Jasmine Heightens spiritual awareness. An aroma favored by angels.

Lavender Helps to integrate spirituality into everyday life.

Myrrh Strengthens spirituality. Builds a bridge between heaven and earth.

Neroli Promotes direct communication with spirit guides.

Rose Promotes a sense of spiritual connection. An aroma favored by angels.

Rosemary Helps us to remember our spiritual path and dedication. Inspires faith.

Rosewood Facilitates opening of the Crown center when one is ready.

Sandalwood Promotes deep meditation. Encourages states of higher consciousness.

Spikenard Increases love for God, higher self, the Divine.

Thyme Restores spiritual fortitude.

Valerian Increases love for the Divine.

Violet Increases spirituality.

COMMON IMBALANCES

Constricted energy:

Apathetic—lavender, lemon, orange, tangerine.

Feelings of isolation and separateness—rose, lavender.

125

Lack of purpose—rose, sandalwood, frankincense.
Fear of death—rosewood, melissa, tangerine.
Life seems senseless—rose, lavender, frankincense.
Congested energy:
Spiritual addiction—rosewood, elemi, frankincense.
Confusion—cedarwood, neroli, geranium, lemon.
Disassociation with body—frankincense, sandalwood, myrrh.

Crown Energy Center Blends

For bringing all the energy centers into balance and unifying them with the Divine:
5 drops frankincense
5 drops lavender
1 T. jojoba oil

For allowing the mind to receive direction and love from the angelic realm:
4 drops rose
4 drops sandalwood
2 drops angelica
1 T. jojoba oil

For integrating spiritual guidance into our daily lives in a grounded way:
6 drops cedarwood
2 drops elemi
2 drops myrrh
1 T. jojoba oil

Using a Pendulum to Assess the Energy Centers

A pendulum can be a useful tool to test the functioning of the energy centers. The swing of a pendulum is not only affected by energy currents, but also demonstrates energy flow, showing in its movement which energy center or centers need assistance. A healthy center sets the pendulum spinning clockwise in a circle. If out-of-balance, the pendulum might either be still, move in the other direction (counter-clockwise), or swing in an odd shape such as an oval or flat-line. Finally, a balanced energy center system would be indicated by the pendulum swinging at relatively the same size for each center. When energy centers are unbalanced, the pendulum swing can be very large, indicating congestion (too much energy) or very small, indicating constriction (too little energy).

A pendulum consists of a weight secured at the end of a string or chain. The chain needs to be long enough (six inches or more) to allow the weight to swing freely. You may purchase a pendulum made of materials such as brass or crystal, but it is just as effective to make one with a piece of thin string and a small weight, such as a button.

127

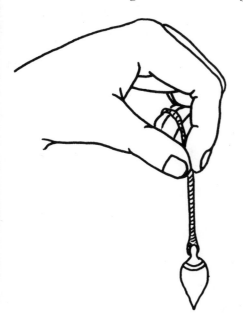

Hold the string or chain of the pendulum so the weight is about three inches away from the body over an energy center. Hold your arm and hand still, and wait for the pendulum to move. The weight will begin to respond to the center's energy field, moving in the circular direction, size, and shape of the energy center, giving you an indication of its condition.

After a Subtle Energy Session

To further the unfolding and deepening of a session, it is helpful to give your receivers an essential oil or blend to take home. Every time he or she smells or applies it, the oil will support the beneficial changes that have occurred during the session, and the fragrance will direct the receiver's memory to the experience and expectation of healing. In this way, the oils are working as a psychological support as well as a vibrational tool.

When at home, the receiver can repeat some of the techniques used during a session to assist energy centers. They can smell the oil from the bottle, or place it on a tissue to inhale when needed or desired. With an anointing oil, they can place a drop under their nose, put a drop on their hands and hold it over an energy center with the intent to balance, or place a drop on their body at the location of the energy center or body area needing help.

You may also suggest visualization techniques that can help your receiver work on their energy centers at home. As they apply the anointing oil or blend, instruct them to:

1. Visualize the energy center's associated color flowing from the essential oil or blend into the center, creating balance and harmony. For example, see a beautiful, sky blue flowing from essential oil of chamomile (German) into the fifth (Throat) center.

2. Visualize the center shining with its clear color, round, open, moving clockwise, looking and being healthy and balanced.

3. Create a meaningful image to represent the center as being strong, healthy and balanced. Some examples include animals, plants, nature scenes, or personally meaningful symbols. Visualize the image being planted in that center, and growing there, bringing wellness. For examples: a bear in the first center; a chamomile plant in the fifth center, an opened, orange rose in the second center, or a peaceful, green meadow for the Heart center.

Affirmations are also powerful tools for helping to balance energy centers. These brief, positive intention statements can be said internally or out loud whenever your receiver smells or applies the oil or blend. Below are some suggested ones, but, as always, tailor these to suit your receiver's needs. Your receiver may also choose to create their own.

Base

I am safe.

I am healthy and strong.

I have all that I need.

I experience abundance in my life.

I am grounded and centered.

Sacral

I celebrate my body and sensuality.

I enjoy my sexuality.

I freely and easily create.

I feel my feelings, and they give me important information about myself
and others.

I invite healthy and supportive relationships into my life.

I experience joy in my life.

Solar Plexus

I appreciate who I am and what I do.

I hold healthy and appropriate boundaries at all times.

I can manifest what I need and want.

I am a person of integrity and courage.

I am confident in my abilities.

Heart

I am love.

I accept and love myself and others.

I am guided by faith and strengthened by hope.

I love my body.

It is safe for me to open myself to giving and receiving love.

Throat

I can speak my truth.

I listen with loving, thoughtful attention.

What I have to say is worthy of being expressed and heard.

I know when to speak and when to be silent.
I have all the time I need.

Third Eye

My mind is clear and focused.
I can trust my intuition.
I open my mind to new ideas, new perspectives.
I can discern what is, for me, the truth.
My mind is clear, calm, and spacious.
I am learning about wisdom.

Crown

I am connected with my spiritual path.
My being is filled with the light of Spirit/God.
I trust in God.
I bring Spirit into my daily life.
Each moment is divine.
I love, and am loved by God/Spirit.

Case Studies with Ruah Bull

Ruah Bull, M.A., co-author of this book, has worked for twenty years in the healing arts as a counselor, hypnotherapist, and energy healer. Following are interesting case studies and excellent examples of what can be done with subtle energy, intention, and essential oils.

1) A man had severe arthritis in his left shoulder, wrist, and hand. I was trying to help him send more energy through his arm, but it was not moving. I put a clearing spray of cedarwood, eucalyptus, and juniper on my hands, and a bit beneath his nose. The energy began to move, and the client reported a wonderful, soothing heat running down his arms. After giving him a blend to use at home and teaching him self-hypnosis to affirm the sensation, he now comes in monthly rather than weekly, and reports with delight that for the first time in years, he has greater movement in his fingers.

2) A student preparing for his acupuncture licensing exams became so worried about failing that he was unable to concentrate, and didn't recall what he was studying. I used the Brain Balance hand position with cedarwood. Afterwards, he felt better prepared to study, and more confident. He was instructed to diffuse rosemary in the room when he studied to promote mental clarity. He received several sessions to help him stop over-worrying, and he reported that the fragrance of cedarwood had become associated with feeling emotionally relaxed and mentally alert. He placed some cedarwood on his wrist before the exam, and smelled it a few times during the exam when he became anxious. He passed both parts of his exam, and now says that he can bring back the effects of the Brain Balance by smelling cedarwood whenever he feels too nervous to be present for one of his patients.

3) An elderly woman living in a nursing home was feeling depressed and apathetic. She reported that she was physically exhausted, and didn't want to get up out of her easy chair or leave her room. I put orange on my hands, placed my hands on her knees as I sat facing her in her chair, and used the Filling technique as we chatted. After about 15 minutes, she reported feeling a bit more energy, and was willing to go to the dining room

131

for her meal. She particularly loved lavender, both for its fragrance and the pleasant memories it brought her. The nursing home staff agreed to spray lavender in her room several times a day, and they reported that her mood greatly improved. They also noted that she seemed to be sleeping more comfortably at night, and they wanted to try aromatherapy with other residents.

4) A deeply spiritual woman was distressed by her need to fire an employee. She was afraid to hurt the person's feelings, but also believed that she had to be truthful about why the person was being released. Just before her meeting with the employee, we made a blend of both German and Roman chamomile, with a drop of bergamot to energize the heart and oakmoss to ground, and used it for Energy Center Balancing. Afterward, she felt able to hold her ground and speak her truth in both a clear, respectful, and compassionate manner. She reported later that although it had still been difficult for her, she had been able to act from her spiritual beliefs, and treat both herself and the other person with dignity and respect. The following week when we met, she was remembering other difficult situations when she had been "attacked" for speaking her truth. We blended rosemary, fennel, and juniper to place on the third energy center. I did a Simple Hold on her third center for about 10 minutes and she released many old feelings that she had taken on from other people—especially their anger—and she reported feeling much lighter than she had in a long time.

5) A woman with pre-menstrual syndrome (PMS) had not been able to find much relief. In a session, we blended rose and jasmine, and worked on her second energy center with a Simple Hold, followed by Energy Center Balancing, using lavender, and then another Simple Hold on the second center. She began to weep after getting in touch with all of the messages she had received as a little girl about menstruation being a curse, and how that had translated into hatred of her female body. She was able to take these issues to her therapist, and by integrating energy work and aromatherapy on her belly (rose and jasmine to support the feminine) and her Heart center (rose and bergamot to promote self-love and love of her body) with her therapy, she was able to experience both a deep psychological healing as well as much relief from her PMS symptoms.

An Exercise

Pick one of the subtle energy hand positions, practice it on a receiver, and notice what happens. What does the receiver experience? What do you experience? Now place an appropriate essential oil or essential oil blend on your hands, and practice the same hand position. What does the receiver notice? What is different from the first exercise? What is the same? What do you notice the second time? Experiment with the different techniques and oils and discover how they complement each other.

Note: It can be helpful to educate your receiver about what it means to notice the effects of a particular oil or technique. Let them know that there may be a change in feeling—a different temperature (hot or cold), or a different sensation (tight, loose, relaxed, hard, blocked, flowing, empty, tingling, heavy, or light). They may perceive a color, texture, or see an image. Some people hear things. Others will not perceive anything at all. Whatever happens for them is right for them at that time. Be supportive, no matter what they experience.

Recommended Reading

Sacred Space: Clearing and Enhancing the Energy of Your Home, Denise Linn (New York: Ballantine Books, 1995).

A Handbook for Light Workers, David Cousins (Dartmouth, England: Barton House, 1993).

Affirmations, Cathy Guiswite (New York: Andrews McMeel Publishing, 1996).

Healing Words, Larry Dossey (San Francisco: Harpers, 1995).

Pendulum Power, Greg Neilsen and Joseph Polansky (New York: Harper Collins, 1987).

S I X

Helping Ourselves

*E*nergy. We want it, and we are drawn to people who radiate it. When we have it, we feel great, and when we don't, we feel as though we're missing out on life. How can we be stewards of our vital energy, cultivating it, and manifesting more when we need it?"
—William Collinge, *Subtle Energy*

Cultivating your own vital energy is necessary to be able to give effective subtle energy sessions because it takes energy to send energy. Energy is gathered, supported, and maintained by taking care of ourselves—nourishing our bodies and souls, prioritizing our time on things that are important, and making positive changes. The energy in our body is not static. It can be increased and strengthened, and it can be depleted. By keeping our energy strong, we have the capacity to be of service to others.

Our Four Dimensions

The level and strength of our energy depends on the vitality of four dimensions that determine our health and wholeness: physical, mental, emotional, and spiritual. It is our responsibility as givers to understand our strengths and weaknesses in these areas so we can build our vital energy and avoid depletion. The description of each dimension below is followed by a few questions. Take the time to answer these questions, ponder your responses, and reflect on their meaning in relationship to your level of energy and how you can improve it. As you build vitality in these four dimensions, your physical as well as subtle bodies are strengthened, increasing your capacity to send healing energy.

137

Physical Well-being

Diet. Primary to physical health is eating wholesome, natural, nourishing food. Buy organic whenever possible, and vary the food you eat. Adopt a philosophy of eating that maximizes good health, but that is also pleasurable. Experiment with different theories such as macrobiotic, vegetarian, lacto-vegetarian, or low-carbohydrate. Pay attention to your energy response. Some people do best on a vegetarian diet, while others need meat occasionally. Food is meant to be enjoyed but avoid over-eating—it strains the digestive system. Be aware of food allergies. They can deplete your energy as well as cause nutrient deficiencies. You may require sup-

plements to attain optimal health. Consider seeing a nutritionist to help you design an eating program that is right for you. Ask yourself: Am I eating the best food for my health? Am I eating consciously? Do I enjoy my food? What can I do to improve my eating habits?

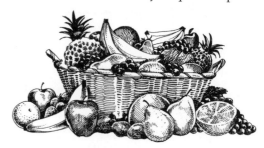

138

Exercise. The human body is designed for action and movement. It wears faster from disuse than it does from use, and operates better with more work than less. Being physically fit is a part of good health. Regular exercise strengthens the heart muscle, increases circulation, makes bones less brittle, improves mental health by promoting clearer thinking and confidence, improves lung function, and makes the body more resilient and

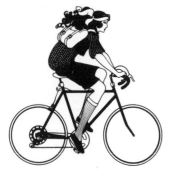

resistant to disease. There is a type of exercise for everyone, whether it be active such as tennis or running, or quiet such as stretching or yoga. Try to include some form of exercise in your everyday routine. What is your form of exercise? How often do you exercise? Do you enjoy it? If not, what can be done to make it more pleasurable? How can you improve your exercise program?

Rest. In the plant and animal world, we see numerous examples of the natural rhythm of activity followed by rest. Bears hunt and eat, and then hibernate. A puppy plays hard, and then collapses and sleeps. A plant that flowers in summer is dormant during winter. Nature teaches us that a balance of rest and activity supports creativity and growth. Wayne Muller, author of *Sabbath: Remembering the Sacred Rhythm of Rest and Delight,* says, "Because we do not rest, we lose our way. We miss the compass points that show us where to go. We lose the nourishment that gives us succor. We miss the quiet that gives us wisdom." Take some time each day for pleasurable rest such as taking a nap, reading a book, watching a little television, or listening to music. Discover what is restful and restorative for you, and give yourself permission to enjoy it. Ask yourself: Do I partake in pleasurable rest everyday? If not, what prevents me? How can I make it a part of my daily routine?

Sleep. Sleep repairs and rejuvenates our bodies and spirits. In order to avoid energetic depletion, you need your optimum amount of sleep

every night. If you are getting enough sleep, you wake up without an alarm, feeling refreshed and revitalized, and ready for the day. The average requirement is eight hours, which can vary with the seasons, or during times of illness and emotional stress. Fill in the following: I get an average of ____ hours of sleep per night.

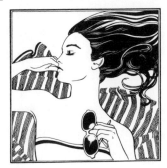

My ideal sleep period is ____ hours. Then answer: If I am not getting enough sleep, what can I do to get more? (Should I go to bed earlier? Can I take a short nap during the day?)

Mental Well-being

Work. Whether it is a paid job, volunteer assignments, or parenting children, our work is one of the most important and time-consuming parts of our lives. It is a major contributor and depletor of our energy, and needs to be in balance with the rest of our life in order for us to feel whole. Love of work is rewarding, satisfying, and builds energy, yet overwork can be depleting. Unrewarding or unenjoyable work can be severely draining, and a change of job may be necessary in order to be healthy. It is particularly important after a rough day at work to take care of yourself to rebuild energy. When work days are good, that alone will help build up reserves. Ask yourself: Is my work enjoyable most of the time? Do I value what I am doing? In what ways is it meaningful to me? How is my energy before, during, and after work? What can I do to make my work situation better?

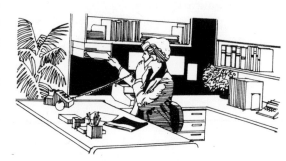

Study. Activities that engage and challenge the mind strengthen our mental and creative capacities. Choose exercises for both sides of your brain—the logical left, and the creative right. Taking classes, doing crossword puzzles, or engaging in stimulating conversation are ways to stretch and energize your logical mind. Exploring the arts, intuitively interpreting your dreams, or letting your imagination play are good for your creative mind. Keep mental activities in balance because overactive minds can deplete energy. Ask yourself: What do I enjoy doing to challenge my logical mind? What do I do to cultivate my creative mind? Which do I enjoy more? Are my mental activities in balance? If not, what can I do to improve them?

Play. Joyful play is important to energize the body and mind, and free the emotions and spirit. It comes quite naturally to children. Play is personal and takes many forms such as engaging in sports, pursuing a hobby, practicing the piano, sewing, spending time with your pets, or dancing to your favorite music. Ask yourself: What do I enjoy as play? How often do I play? How can I bring more playfulness into my life?

Emotional Well-being

Your emotional life includes the sum total of all your relationships, an accumulation of past and present experiences—primarily with people but

140

also with those situations that are a source of self-love and self-esteem such as work, hobbies, and personal goals. Supporting and balancing your emotional life helps you to remain energized. Out-of-balance emotions can drain your energy and take a toll on your health. Emotions are powerful and complex, and can be both constructive and destructive. For example, love, compassion, and joy build energy and expand the auric field. Hate, jealousy, and fear deplete energy and decrease the auric field.

Tending to your emotions involves learning how to recognize and acknowledge your true feelings, and then being able to express them in a positive way. Some people are more extroverted, and need to talk openly about their feelings. Others are more introverted, and need to be private. Sometimes we need help in learning to identify and express emotions. There are many competent professionals, as well as devoted friends that can help with this process.

Pay particular attention to the people in your life. Healthy relation-

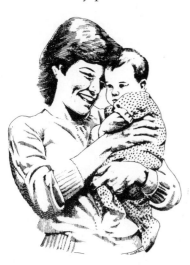

ships are a balance of giving and receiving. Distance yourself from people who are abusive or emotionally draining. If this is not possible, establish boundaries and fill your physical and subtle bodies with positive, grounded energy so there is no room for negativity. Examine your relationships with your mother, father, siblings, children, friends, spouse, neighbors, and co-workers. Think about how they may energize or deplete you. Ask yourself: How is my energy different with different people? What relationships make me feel good? Which ones drain me? What activities do I do with people that make me feel good? Am I spending enough time with the people I love? How can I improve my relationships?

Our emotional life is also sustained by those things that support a healthy sense of self-esteem and self-love. This can be many things such as

141

building a cabinet, teaching a child something new, winning a race, breaking an unwanted habit, learning something new, or helping others. Ask yourself: What experiences in my life do I value? What brings me a sense of emotional fulfillment? What unhealthy habits would I like to stop? What goals have I accomplished? What goals would I still like to accomplish?

As you learn to support and experience emotional well-being, your energy system strengthens. Being present with your feelings and in your relationships builds your energy and allows you to be more fully with your receivers and their emotions when giving a session.

Spiritual Well-being

Everybody has a spiritual dimension—it is a natural part of being human. Spirituality is, at heart, the place where we connect to that which is greater than ourselves. For some, this means praying to God, meditating, or chanting to the Great Spirit. For others, it means hiking in nature, or being involved with charities that serve mankind.

142

Worldly success is often measured by our vocation, family life, wealth, or fame. Yet, there are many outwardly successful people who feel empty and wonder why they are not happy. This is an example, energetically, of a depleted seventh energy center—our center for spirituality.

Traditionally, our spiritual nature has been nurtured by attending church, meditation groups, nature ceremonies, or through sacred dance and song. However, there are other profound, non-religious ways to strengthen spirituality such as working in a garden, or being inspired by great art, music, and literature. For many, giving and receiving energy healing, and working with essential oils is a spiritual experience.

As your spiritual connection grows, everything you do and experience can strengthen your well-being on this level. Washing the dishes becomes a prayer, gardening an act of worship, and doing the laundry an act of contemplation and gratitude. Along with the practices and ceremonies we set aside as sacred, there grows an illuminating sense that even the most mundane act can be holy. As the seventh energy center draws that light into your being, your entire auric field is infused with brilliance, and you can give—to yourself and others—without depletion. Ask yourself: What is holy to me? How would I describe my relationship to spirit? What in my life supports my spiritual well-being? Is there anything that I would like to add to my spiritual practice?

We all have these four dimensions in our lives. They must be well tended in order to maintain health and well-being: physical, mental, emotional, and spiritual. Review each of these and make a list of things you would like to change. Pick one, note how you are going to introduce this change, and allow yourself two months in which to accomplish it. At the end of each week, assess your progress. If you have been successful, how was it able to happen? If not, what prevented it from happening? Was your goal realistic? If so, what will you do so that it can be accomplished next week? If not, how can you change your goal to make it realistic? Repeat this process at the end of each week.

Keep in mind that perfectionism drains energy. Do the best you can, be realistic about your goals, and start slowly. It usually takes two to three months for a new habit to become solidly entrenched. After a month or two of enjoying your new habit, pick another change from your list, and go through the same process. Notice how the change has affected other areas of your life, and look forward to enjoying a new level of well-being.

Self-Care Questionnaire

Self-care is the foundation of a nurturing, supportive relationship with ourselves. We acknowledge the need to be our own true friend, tending to the child within us, and fulfilling our requirements for play, sleep, nourishing food, companionship, and love. Subtle energy therapy emphasizes the need for self-care so that we have enough energy to be able to draw healing energy into our bodies, and send it out through our hands and auric field. One goal of self-care is to build and maintain energy so that we are able to give.

Many givers find it a challenge to be as kind to themselves as they are to others. Before you begin offering subtle energy sessions to friends, family, or clients, examine your thoughts and feelings about receiving and the idea of self-care. Answer the following questions and reflect upon your answers.

Receiving

1. Generally, am I comfortable or uncomfortable about receiving help from others?
2. What are the situations in which I feel comfortable? Why?
3. Are there particular people from whom I am comfortable receiving help? Why?
4. What are the situations in which I feel uncomfortable receiving help? Why?
5. Are there particular people from whom I am uncomfortable receiving help? Why?
6. What is selfishness?
7. What is generosity?
8. When is helping someone else actually being selfish?
9. When is refusing to receive help an act of selfishness?

Self-care
1. What does self-care mean to me? How do I feel about it?
2. What do I already do to take care of myself?
3. What are the things that I am not doing? Why?
4. Who supports me in my efforts to take care of myself? How?
5. Who is not supportive? How?
6. How can I start taking better care of myself? When?

Taking Time / Making Time

In a recent interview in *Sounds True Catalogue* (Summer 1999), writer Wayne Muller quoted Thomas Merton, "To allow ourselves to be carried away by a multitude of conflicting concerns, to surrender to too many demands, to commit oneself to too many projects, to want to help everyone in everything, is to succumb to violence." Merton believes that when we are busy all the time, even busy with good things, the frenzy "kills the root of inner wisdom." Even though we are trying to do good work, if we are desperate, rushed, and frantic, we will unintentionally create suffering for people.

Most people's lives are very busy and the desire to take care of ourselves is often thwarted by not being able to find the time. Self-care may require a re-shuffling of priorities, cutting back on responsibilities, and striving to simply do less. We are worth the effort. Completing the following exercise will help you prioritize how you spend your time, making more time available for things that build your energy.

1. Make a list of all the things you spend time doing.
2. Now separate this list into 3 parts, A, B, and C, and assign your daily, weekly, or monthly schedule to each item in each list.
   A. Top priorities. These are the most important things to you that need to be accomplished. It might be food shopping, work, cooking, exercise at the gym, or paying bills.
   B. Second priorities. These are important but not as important as items in A. For example: Doing the laundry, cleaning the house, writing letters, reading, or clothes shopping.
   C. Lowest priorities. These are things that are not so important but notice that some of the things on this list can move up to B or A if put off for another time, such as washing the dogs or mowing the lawn.
3. Look at your C list. Is there anything you would be willing to change? For example, could you read just the Sunday paper and not the daily? Could you plant a garden that requires less care?

4. Look at your B list. Is there anything that can be moved to list C or be done in an easier way?

5. Look at your A list. Is there anything that can be moved to list B or be done in an easier way?

6. Now, place your name above each of the three lists. What self-care practices are on your A list per day, week, and month. Your B list? Your C list?

7. If there aren't any or just a few, it's time to insert self-care activities into all three lists that support the four dimensions of well-being on a daily, weekly, and monthly basis. Think about adding a monthly massage, a daily walk, and a weekly dinner out.

Helpful Daydreams

To integrate self-care practices, and make changes in your life, a simple and common visualization technique, similar to daydreaming, can assist you in programming yourself. When you make an improvement in one area of your life, it affects other areas as well.

Get comfortable, close your eyes, and take some relaxing breaths.

In your imagination, experience making a change and taking care of yourself in a new way, such as exercising regularly. See yourself, feel yourself doing this. Watch yourself as if you were on a movie screen, then step into the movie and be there.

Bring in all of your senses. What do you see? How do you feel? Are there any sounds that you can hear? Are there any fragrances, or even tastes?

Let this experience become as clear and real as possible, knowing that you are now positively programming yourself. When you have practiced and integrated changes in your life internally this way, it becomes easier to manifest them outwardly.

148

Optional. If there is an essential oil that relates to and supports your desired change (such as lavender for relaxation, frankincense for meditation, rosemary for mental clarity, pine for physical energy) you can smell that oil during this exercise, and give yourself the suggestion that each time you smell this scent it becomes easier and more natural for you to practice your self-care behavior. In this way, the oil becomes an anchor, and can assist you in making this change.

Nourishment Through the Senses

Rosalyn Bruyere believes, "The only thing that affects our body is the level and kind of energy to which it is exposed." She further explains, "If we are exposed to negative energies of any kind long enough, the potential result will be detrimental to our health—physical, emotional, mental, or spiritual." Logically, then, the opposite is true. If we are exposed to positive energy long enough, the results are beneficial. One can see how important it is for our good health and well-being to pay attention to what we come in contact with, especially through our five senses: taste, touch, sight, hearing, and smell—the doorways to our physiological, psychological, and spiritual make-up. Ideally, we would live in a beautiful, natural setting amidst trees and flowers, eat nourishing food, hear lovely sounds, experience beautiful aromas, and spend time with wonderful people.

The five senses can be used in a positive way:

Taste. Not only is it important to eat whole, natural food, it is also important to enjoy it, and experience a variety of flavors. Ayurveda teaches that there are six different tastes, each of which we should encounter every day to stimulate different parts of the brain. They are: sweet (e.g., bread, honey), sour (e.g. yogurt, lemon), salty (e.g. pickles, soy sauce), bitter (e.g. spinach, endive), astringent (e.g. beans, pomegranate), and pungent (e.g. pepper, ginger).

149

Touch. Human beings need to be touched for good health. The skin is replete with nerve endings that stimulate and send messages to the brain. Hugs and hand-holds help us feel connected, and provide emotional nourishment. Massage is especially beneficial, combining both human touch and muscle manipulation to soothe, relax, and relieve pain.

Sight. Color and light travel through the eye via the retina to the hypothalamus in the brain, affecting our endocrine system and emotions. Color has been used therapeutically throughout history because our bodies and minds respond to it. For example, red is energizing, blue is relaxing, and green is balancing. Having things at home and in the workplace that are visually pleasing in both color and design supports our well-being.

Hearing. Music was an integral part of ancient Egyptian medicine, and the Greeks believed that music restored health to both body and soul. It is thought that certain types of music (generally soft and soothing tones) cause the body to release endorphins that can relieve pain and induce relaxation. Music can also be used to energize and uplift. Interestingly, silence is also therapeutic. Anthropologist Angeles Arien says that in many indigenous tribes the healer will ask an ill person four questions, one of which is, "When did you lose your love of the sweet territory of silence?" Silence is the sound of the seventh energy center, and can be very rejuvenating—a welcome respite from a noisy world.

Smell. As we have seen, aromas affect us on many levels. When odor molecules enter our nose, they affect the limbic system in the brain, causing physiological and psychological responses. Aromatherapy uses natural fragrances to relax, relieve stress and anxiety, ease depression, and energize. In addition, an aroma that has wonderful associations, such as a particular food cooking, can be aromatically beneficial.

Are Your Energy Centers Healthy?

Our energy anatomy (energy centers and subtle bodies) reflects our state of well-being. As givers, we need to keep abreast of the imbalances in our own energy centers. Completing the following questionnaire will give you an idea as to which centers may be out of balance. Answering yes to four or more of the questions associated with an energy center indicates an imbalance.

Energy Center Questionnaire
FIRST/BASE

Do you feel disassociated from your body?

Are you overweight?

Are you underweight?

Do you have a weak physical constitution?

Does life on earth feel like a burden?

Are you fearful?

Are you disorganized?

Are you possessive and/or materialistic?

Are you worried about financial security?

Are you accident prone?

SECOND/SACRAL

Do you suppress your sexual desires?

Do you have a negative attitude about sex?

Does sexuality make you nervous?

Do you lack passion or excitement about life?

Are you emotionally dependent?

Does your creativity feel blocked?

Do you feel guilty?

Are you afraid of making a commitment?

Are you obsessed with sexual thoughts or feelings?

151

THIRD/SOLAR PLEXUS

Do you have low energy?

Do you have low self-esteem?

Are you weak willed?

Are you easily upset or discouraged?

Do you feel ashamed of who you are?

Are you unreliable?

Are you manipulative and controlling?

Are you unable to relax?

Do you have temper outbursts?

Are you stubborn?

Are you prone to digestive problems?

Do you always like to be in control?

Are you afraid of rejection?

FOURTH/HEART

Are you anti-social?

Are you intolerant of others?

Do you have a fear of intimacy?

Are you overly sensitive?

Are you depressed?

Are you experiencing grief?

Are you indifferent?

Do you have a jealous nature?

Do you have difficulty breathing?

Do you take care of others but not yourself?

FIFTH/THROAT

Do you have a fear of speaking?

Do you have a weak voice?

Are you unable to express your true feelings?

Are you shy or withdrawn?

Do you speak harshly to others?

Do you talk too much?
Do you tell lies?
Are you unable to listen to others?
Do you frequently have a sore throat?
Do you feel you have nothing worthwhile to say?
Do you clench your jaw or grind your teeth?

SIXTH/THIRD EYE

Are you out of touch with reality?
Do you have a poor memory?
Are you forgetful?
Do you feel confused?
Do you have impaired vision?
Do you have difficulty concentrating?
Do you have nightmares?
Do you often misunderstand situations?
Do you have frequent headaches?
Are you over-analytical?
Do you doubt your intuition?

153

SEVENTH/CROWN

Are your apathetic?
Do you feel lonely or isolated?
Do you feel you have no purpose in life?
Are you afraid of dying?
Does life seems senseless?
Are you over-attached to your belongings or relationships?
Do you have an addictive relationship with spirituality?
Do you search for answers outside yourself?

Positive Actions to Strengthen the Energy Centers

ROOT. Take care of yourself. Maintain a weight that is healthy for you. Rest, eat well, and exercise. Do work you love. Develop a conscious relationship with money. Organize.

SACRAL. Give and receive. Create. Play. Experience balanced sexuality.

SOLAR PLEXUS. Accomplish a goal. Learn to relax. Be proud of who you are.

HEART. Give love and compassion unconditionally. Be patient with yourself and others. Breathe deeply.

THROAT. Speak the truth. Speak gently. Sing or chant. Listen well. Take time.

THIRD EYE. Visualize. Imagine. Intuit. Close your eyes and feel the sun entering this center.

CROWN. See the Divine in everybody, everywhere. Look inside for answers.

Constricting Feelings Associated with the Energy Centers

Energy center researchers such as Anodea Judith have described each energy center as having associated feelings or mental states that especially constrict its energy, throwing it out of balance. The chart below has been the most useful to the authors and indicates these relationships.

ENERGY CENTER	CONSTRICTING FEELINGS
First (Base)	Fear
Second (Sacral)	Guilt
Third (Solar)	Shame
Fourth (Heart)	Grief
Fifth (Throat)	Selfishness
Sixth (Third Eye)	Closed mindedness
Seventh (Crown)	Over-attachment

154

Our sense of health and wholeness depends, in part, on being able to feel, and then properly deal with those feelings. From this perspective, no feelings, including fear, guilt, shame, or grief, are bad or wrong. Each of these emotions can be a healthy signal. Fear alerts us to situations that may be dangerous. Guilt and shame can provide the impetus to change our behavior or make amends. Grief is the natural response to loss—a part of the heart's healing process.

However, each of these feelings also has an unhealthy manifestation. This can be the result of being unable to fully feel, unable to move through the feeling, and especially being unable to become free of it. When fear is immobile, one may become fearful about change or about life itself. When guilt or shame is immobile, a debilitating self-hatred may emerge. Grief, unprocessed, can transform into depression or bitterness. Selfishness, untended, can destroy the capacity for relationships. Rigid, close-mindedness diminishes creativity, and over-attachment can lead to addictions.

Healthy feelings are distinguished from unhealthy feelings by their movement as we experience them. Emotion is e-motion—energy in motion. Does your fear immobilize you, or are you able to use it to create more safety, security and trust? Does your guilt or shame paralyze you into believing that you are unworthy, or assist you in determining to be a better and more loving human being? Does your grief permanently shut down your heart, or help you realize the preciousness of life—the gifts of this tender, fleeting existence? Does your selfishness finally help you listen to yourself so you can hear others? Does becoming aware of your close-mindedness help you discern what you truly believe and also be willing to examine those beliefs? Does feeling how over-attachment shuts down the life force help you open yourself to life's experiences? Healthy feelings may move slowly, sometimes almost imperceptibly, but there is sense of aliveness as we pass through the phases of the experience.

Special Techniques to Tend to the Energy Centers and Auric Field
Very warm bath. Use one cup of apple cider vinegar, or one cup of mineral salts or Epsom salts to neutralize negative energy and balance the auric field. After the bath, let all the water out of the tub, and rinse thoroughly with warm water while scrubbing with a loofah or washcloth to remove any residue. End with a cool water rinse, towel dry, dress, and then rest for one to two hours while sipping room temperature water (two to four cups).

Shower. After a shower, while your skin in still wet, put 4 drops of cedarwood, juniper, rosemary, vetiver, or lavender in the palms of your hands and quickly apply, evenly, to your entire body to clear and cleanse the auric field.

Note: Showers and baths are recommended on the day after having a subtle energy session, so as not to disrupt the newly established energy pattern.

Energy workouts. Yoga, qi gong, and tai chi help to balance the energy centers and build energy.

A subtle energy session. Giving or receiving a subtle energy session helps to balance and strengthen the energy centers and auric field.

Sing or chant. Singing and chanting helps to mobilize and balance the first through the fifth energy centers.

Sound. Drumming, using rattles, or shaking bells around your auric field helps to cleanse and balance.

Being present. Sitting with a favorite tree, rock, plant, animal, or person will help balance the energy centers through the heart center.

Create. Make something beautiful, especially with mirrors, bells, color, and/or feathers. These are things that move and balance energy.

Smudge. Burning cleansing herbs such as sage or juniper and waving the smoke around your body helps to cleanse the auric field.

Recommended Reading

Hypnosis for Change, Josie Hadley and Carol Staudacher (Oakland, CA: New Harbinger Publishing, 1991).

Buffalo Woman Comes Singing, Brooke Medicine Eagle (New York: Ballantine Books, 1991).

Subtle Energy, William Collinge, Ph.D. (New York: Warner Books, 1998).

Sevenfold Journey, Anodea Judith & Selene Vega (Freedom, CA: Crossing Press, 1993).

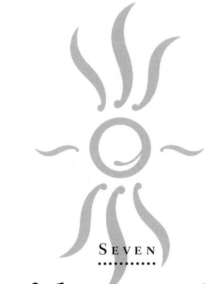

SEVEN

Helping Others

When you give a subtle energy session to someone, whether it is a family member, a friend, or a client, you have certain ethical responsibilities. The task for givers is to create a safe and protected place in which to give a session; to be in a positive, loving state of mind; to be open to the healing energy of the universe; and to establish a respectful, caring, and helpful relationship with the receiver. The following guidelines foster this healing relationship.

Remember: the healer is within the receiver. Your role as giver is to facilitate a process, not to "fix" the receiver, or expect a certain outcome. The body/mind wisdom of the receiver will use what you provide in the best way possible. Your intention is to be of the most beneficial service to your receiver. Allow energy and the receiver's innate healing ability to do the rest.

Avoid judgement and blame. It is not appropriate to judge or blame someone for what they are experiencing. Shaming the receiver is counterproductive and constricts their energy field. It also does not support the compassionate qualities of the giver's Heart center. Telling someone they have a headache because they "shouldn't have eaten chocolate" or they "need to release anger" is inappropriate, judgmental, and may be entirely wrong. Accept, without judgement, the condition of the receiver.

Confidentiality is necessary to establish trust between giver and receiver. Never discuss what happens in a session with anyone else, unless it is a professional supervisor. This includes the receiver. For example, if your receiver is a friend that you see regularly, recognize that the subtle energy session is a special and separate occasion. Do not casually refer to it outside of that time, unless they choose to discuss it.

Respect the receiver's limits. People have different comfort levels concerning physical touch and emotional sharing. Not every receiver wants a hug from you. Not everyone wants to talk in depth about their present symptoms, or about themselves. Part of creating a safe and protected place is to let the receiver know that you recognize and honor their boundaries.

We recommend that a subtle energy session be given with as little dialogue as possible. Especially, keep your personal sharing to a minimum. Share, without judgement, only when it will make the other person know that you understand and can empathize with them. A session is his or her time to receive. If, however, the receiver feels the need to talk, it may be a part of their healing process. In this case, be a good listener.

Active Listening

In order to be an effective giver, we must first be a good listener. It is a great gift to offer your receiver the remarkable experience of being truly and fully heard. For many, it is healing in itself. An active listener is someone who listens closely, acknowledges what they hear, and pays attention to the following.

Body language. While someone is talking, if we turn our back to them, refuse to make eye contact, or are busy doing something else, we have sent body language signals that we are not paying attention. Situate yourself at a comfortable distance from the receiver, face them, and occasionally make eye contact. Be calm and comfortable. This signals your receiver that you are present and interested.

Paraphrasing. Occasionally, repeat back to the receiver what you have heard. For example, "Let me tell you what I've heard you say, and you can tell me if I've understood." This lets the receiver know you are listening, and gives them an opportunity to correct any misunderstandings. It can be helpful as well as reassuring.

Ask open-ended questions. Do not assume that you know what the receiver is experiencing with comments such as, "That must have been hard for you," or "You must have been really angry." In fact, it may not have been hard for them, or they may not have been angry. Instead, ask open-ended questions such as, "How did you feel?" or "What was that like for you?" This allows for a deeper sharing of their experience.

Misplaced empathy. Do not assume you know someone's experience because you had a similar one. Avoid statements such as, "I know exactly what you are going through." Most people resent this comment because, in truth, you do not know—everyone experiences life differently. However, sometimes this type of sharing can be helpful in making the person feel not so alone. "I've had bad sinus headaches, too, and they can be really painful." Share enough to let the person know that you're sympathetic, but then go back to listening closely to them.

Giving advice: As a rule of thumb, only give advice when asked, and always put it in an appropriate, personalized perspective. Unless you are professionally licensed to give particular advice, keeping it personal allows you to share knowledge without claiming inappropriate authority. For example, "This is what works for me . . ." or "Many people have found this helpful . . .."

Appropriate referrals. Become familiar with professionals in your area who deal with problems your receivers may have. This could include medical and psychological professionals as well as complementary care practitioners. When giving referrals, offer at least three choices so your receiver can find the practitioner that suits them best.

Giving a Subtle Energy Session

It is appropriate to offer a subtle energy session whenever a receiver would like one and you have the time, energy, and a balanced state of mind to give one. People receive sessions for all sorts of reasons—physical symptoms, emotional upset, a desire for deep relaxation, a need for energizing, or the comfort of safe touch. We believe the intelligence of the receiver's physical and subtle bodies instructs the energy coming through the giver's hands to be of the quality that is needed, and will be of the most benefit.

The following are descriptions of eight different subtle energy sessions designed for different purposes. Each session lasts for approximately thirty minutes. For children, seniors, or someone who is ill, the session is usually much shorter—about ten minutes. In each session, preparing for and ending the session are the same.

Preparation

Whether you have a special place in which you give subtle energy sessions, or you use whatever space is available, always take a few moments to clear, cleanse, and set sacred space. For example, spray the room with a blend of equal parts cedarwood, juniper, and eucalyptus to gently clear and cleanse the area. Use a diffuser to disperse essential oils in the air that support healing such as lavender, rose, rosewood, or palmarosa.

After you have done the initial exercises, "Center in Your Breath" and "Prepare Your Hands" (Chapter 4), you are ready to begin. First, relax your body, your facial muscles and especially the muscles around your eyes. Your visual focus then becomes soft, diffused, and expanded. This helps create a more intuitive and receptive state of mind.

Put a drop of a grounding oil, such as vetiver or patchouli, on your feet. Then put a drop of lavender on your hands to open them to healing energy as you say a simple prayer to attract the most beneficial energy, out loud or silently. A favorite is "May I and this person be healed and filled with light." Always be clear about your intention for the session.

Invite the receiver into the dedicated space, and if you haven't already discussed what it is they want, take a few minutes to do that now,

165

using your active listening skills. This helps you and your receiver focus on what is needed at this time. Ask the receiver to lie down. A massage table is ideal but a bed, table, or the floor, will also work. Whatever it is, be sure that both of you are comfortable. Some people like a pillow under both their neck and knees for support. Cover them with a sheet, and a blanket, if necessary. Encourage them to let you know if they become too hot or too cold so you can remove or add blankets. Healing energy often changes the temperature of the body. You are now ready to give a subtle energy session.

Be considerate in your approach to your receiver, as well as during your departure. Because auric fields extend several inches to several feet beyond the skin, contact is made as soon as the giver's and receiver's bodies are close to each other—before actual physical contact. Abrupt or harsh subtle body connections are disagreeable and jarring. Be calm and gentle. When you are finished with the session, disconnect and leave the auric field the same way, slowly and gently, with respect.

The essential oils used in the following sessions are applied as anointing oils, unless otherwise mentioned. To make an anointing oil use five to ten drops of essential oil in one tablespoon of carrier oil; see Chapter 5 for further details.

A Session for Relaxation and Stress Relief

Open Toes. One to two minutes. Put lavender and/or chamomile on your hands to help your receiver relax and be receptive to the session.

Head Hold. Five minutes. Move quietly to the head. Add a drop of sandalwood to your hands, and rest the receiver's head in your hands. Visualize all stress gently falling away, and being absorbed by the earth. Breathe slowly and deeply. The rhythm of your breath helps the receiver to relax.

Forehead Spread. Three minutes. Continue to use the sandalwood. Imagine that a blue, relaxing light is moving out of your fingers, through the receiver's body, and out their fingers and toes.

Windshield Wipers. Two to three minutes. Use pine to support and strengthen the energy if there is physical exhaustion. Use essential oil of orange to uplift and move stagnant energy if there is mental or emotional exhaustion. Use both, if appropriate. Visualize any remaining stress being gently rocked away, as the body fills with relaxation.

Simple Hold. Two to four minutes. Add a drop of a grounding oil to your hands such as vetiver or cedarwood. Move your hands to gently hold the ankles, and send healing energy for one to two minutes. Then move your hands to the bottoms of the feet, and send energy for another one to two minutes. Imagine that the physical body is deeply relaxed, that all the energy centers are balanced and in harmony with one another, and that the subtle bodies are gently glowing with health and peace.

Sweep and Comb. Two minutes. Mist your receiver with lavender or rose, and gently sweep and comb their auric field.

Close Toes. Two minutes. With lavender on your hands, touch each toe, beginning with the smallest and move up to the big toes. Visualize the energy centers closing to the size that will be best for your receiver during the rest of their day.

A Session for Energizing

Open Toes. One to two minutes. Put lavender and/or chamomile on your hands to help your receiver relax and be receptive to the session.

Head Hold. Five minutes. Use lavender to gently prepare the body to receive energy as you visualize a lavender light coming from your hands and filling first the head, then the spine, and then the rest of the body.

Filling. Three minutes. Put pine on your hands to increase energy in the physical and subtle bodies, and then place them on your receiver's shoulders. Visualize their body and auric field glowing with an energizing light—red, orange, or yellow.

Windshield Wipers. Two to three minutes. Use myrrh to help release any feelings of being immobilized and to increase a sense of movement and flexibility. Visualize a clear red light moving from your hands, up the legs, and into the first energy center.

Energy Ball. Two minutes. Place orange essential oil on you hands to direct a joyful energy into the solar plexus. Visualize the second energy cen-

167

ter glowing in a clear orange and the third in a clear yellow. Place the energy ball over the stomach and let it be absorbed to the degree it can be absorbed.

Grounding Wave. Two minutes. Put patchouli on your hands to connect the subtle and physical bodies, and allow the physical body to integrate the energy in a grounded, balanced way.

Energy Center Balancing. Seven minutes. The receiver turns onto their stomach. Place lavender on your hands to assist in supporting all of the now-energized centers to become balanced with one another. Visualize each center filled with its own color, round, equal in size, and spinning together.

Sweep and Comb. Two minutes. The receiver turns onto their back again. Mist your receiver with lavender or rose, and gently sweep and comb their auric field.

Close Toes. Two minutes. With lavender on your hands, touch each toe, beginning with the smallest and move up to the big toes. Visualize the energy centers closing to the size that will be best for your receiver during the rest of their day.

A Session for Feeling Safe and Secure

Open Toes. One to two minutes. Put lavender and/or chamomile on your hands to help your receiver relax and be receptive to the session.

Head Hold. Five minutes. Place frankincense on your hands, and imagine gently connecting the first and seventh centers with a warm, golden light. Allow your breath to deepen, and visualize your receiver safely held in your hands.

Forehead Spread. Three minutes. With sandalwood on your hands, rest your fingers on their forehead, and send a deep indigo light into the sixth center and a lavender light into the seventh. Visualize that the mind is becoming relaxed and comfortable.

Grounding. Three minutes. Moving to the feet, place vetiver on your hands to help ground. Imagine the receiver fully in their body with a warm, golden, protective seal around the auric field.

Simple Hold. Two minutes. Using myrrh, hold your hands off the body six to twelve inches over the base center. Send a clear red light into the center, and imagine it filling with that light, and becoming balanced and strong. You might imagine a red butterfly opening its wings, or a red rose bud unfolding.

Filling. Two minutes. Put orange essential oil on your hands for joyful energy, and then place your hands on your receiver's feet or shoulders. Gently send a golden light. Let it fill the whole body.

Cleansing Spin. Three minutes. Use lavender to allow any fears or other negative feelings to release fully from the physical body and auric field. Visualize the body inside of a large, beautiful white or lavender ball of energy.

Simple Hold. Two minutes. Return to the feet with vetiver on your hands. Imagine that the ball of energy is now filling with grounding, earth energy. The color may be red or green.

Sweep and Comb. Two minutes. Mist your receiver with lavender or rose, and gently sweep and comb their auric field.

Close Toes. Two minutes. With lavender on your hands, touch each toe, beginning with the smallest and moving up to the big toes. Visualize the energy centers closing to the size that will be best for your receiver during the rest of their day.

A Session for Enhancing Creativity

Open Toes. One to two minutes. Put lavender and/or chamomile on your hands to help your receiver relax and be receptive to the session.

Head Hold. Three minutes. Use cedarwood on your hands to gently release all mental blocks. Visualize the spine in perfect alignment, and each center opening to make contact with creative forces.

Forehead Spread. Two minutes. Place rosemary on your hands. Imagine the sixth center in a clear indigo color, and that the mind is both clear and receptive.

Brain Balance. Five minutes. Lavender oil used during this technique allows clarity and receptivity to direct information and wisdom into the other centers. Visualize the brain in a clear lavender color, and let that lavender flow down through the body bringing it into perfect balance.

Simple Hold. Four positions, one and a half minutes for each position. First, place jasmine on your hands and do a Simple Hold over the second energy center. Visualize this center capable of generating and holding passion and excitement. Let an orange flower bloom here. Then, a drop of pine on the third energy center to strengthen confidence, visualizing a golden sun. Next, using bergamot, move your hands to the fourth center, and visualize a pink, rose, or green flower opening. Imagine any energy block gently melting beneath your hands. Finally, with German chamomile, do a Simple Hold over the fifth center. As a beautiful blue flower opens, imagine the center filled with warmth, energy, and light.

Cleansing Spin. Three minutes. At the head, begin the cleansing spin by putting juniper on your hands, and then placing your hands on the shoulders of your receiver. The spin will help release any negative self-concepts that have stood in the way of full, creative expression.

Energy Center Balancing. Five minutes. The receiver turns onto their stomach. Use geranium on your hands to assist balancing and create relaxed spontaneity.

Sweep and Comb. Two minutes. The receiver turns onto their back again. Mist your receiver with lavender or rose, and gently sweep and comb their auric field.

Close Toes. Two minutes. With lavender on your hands, touch each toe, beginning with the smallest and moving up to the big toes. Visualize the energy centers closing to the size that will be best for your receiver during the rest of their day.

A Session for Confidence and Self-Esteem

Open Toes. One to two minutes. Put lavender and/or chamomile on your hands to help your receiver relax and be receptive to the session.

Head Hold. Two minutes. Elemi creates peace and lucidity, and supports a connection between mind and body. Visualize this mental state as a lavender light fills first the head and then the entire body.

Forehead Spread. Two minutes. To complete the mental balancing, use lavender to support a perfect blend of relaxation and energy. This balance clears the mind so that the receiver can experience the realistic self-awareness that forms the basis of healthy self-esteem.

Windshield Wipers. Two to three minutes. Placing myrrh on the hands, imagine any feelings of immobilization releasing from the body. Then placing hands on the knees, send the intention that your receiver can stand firm yet move forward with confidence.

Simple Hold. Two minutes. Use petitgrain on your hands, and place them over the third center. This promotes self-esteem and the ability to comfortably and confidently be oneself. Imagine this area filling with a clear, golden color—like the sun in its warmth and light.

Cleansing Spin. Three minutes. Using juniper on your hands as they rest on the receiver's shoulders will assist in releasing any negative self-concepts that are ready to be released.

Grounding Wave. Five minutes. Holding the feet, use vetiver to ground your receiver as well as seal and protect the auric field so your receiver's confidence and self-esteem will not be damaged by other people's opinions.

Sweep and Comb. Two minutes. Mist your receiver with lavender or rose, and gently sweep and comb their auric field.

Close Toes. Two minutes. With lavender on your hands, touch each toe, beginning with the smallest and moving up to the big toes. Visualize the energy centers closing to the size that will be best for your receiver during the rest of their day.

A Session for a Joyful Heart

Open Toes. One to two minutes. Put lavender and/or chamomile on your hands to help your receiver relax and be receptive to the session.

Head Hold. Three minutes. Use sandalwood to support all the energy centers, and to open the heart for deep healing. Imagine a glowing white or gold light filling the body.

Grounding Wave. Two minutes. Vetiver grounds, protects, and supports the receiver as they open to the joy of life. Imagine a green, auric cocoon providing a safe container for a joyful heart.

171

Windshield Wipers. Two to three minutes. Orange essential oil used here supports the capacity to experience joy. Then place tangerine on your hands, and touch the receiver's knees, letting the body continue to become full of life and love. Visualize a soft, clear orange or rose light filling the body.

Simple Hold. Two minutes. Place ylang ylang on one hand, holding the second center to release fear and draw in self-esteem. Place rose on your other hand, holding the fourth center to support the Heart on all levels—physical, emotional, mental, and spiritual. Visualize these centers as healthy, strong and clear, and wait until you feel a sense that they are both connected and balanced with each other.

Cleansing Spin. Three minutes. Use lavender on your hands as the cleansing white light surrounds the body to release old, negative emotional patterns, and clear the astral body, allowing deep, life-affirming joy to be integrated emotionally.

Energy Center Balancing. Five minutes. Continuing with the lavender on your hands, visualize each center filling with the potential of joy and love. Perhaps you would like to use the image of a rose, traditionally a symbol of love, opening in each center.

Sweep and Comb. Two minutes. Turning onto their back again, mist your receiver with lavender or rose, and gently sweep and comb their auric field.

Close Toes. Two minutes. With lavender on your hands, touch each toe, beginning with the smallest and moving up to the big toes. Visualize the energy centers closing to the size that will be best for your receiver during the rest of their day.

A Session for Positive Communication

Open Toes. One to two minutes. Put lavender and/or chamomile on your hands to help your receiver relax and be receptive to the session.

Head Hold. Three minutes. Cedarwood disperses energy blockages that prevent your receiver from knowing what they want to say, as well as being able to say it in a positive manner. Imagine a clear lavender or gold light filling first the head, then the body, clearing any blockages.

Forehead Spread. Two minutes. Rosemary creates clarity of thought and perception as well as protection. Imagine the sixth and seventh centers open and spinning, and visualize the auric field as a clear, protective egg whose boundaries prevent your receiver from being confused or unbalanced by other people's thoughts, words, or actions.

Windshield Wiper. Two to three minutes. This assists the body to integrate the increased clarity and awareness. Sandalwood helps to both ground and promote the most positive thoughts, intentions, and words.

Simple Hold. Two minutes. Use essential oil of orange on one of your hands. Rest it on the second energy center to support a deepening trust in life and relationships. On your other hand, place German chamomile, then rest it on the fifth energy center to facilitate the healthy expression of truth. Send balancing energy into each—orange light into the second and blue into the fifth. Hold this position until you sense that the two centers are both connected and balanced with each other. This hold will assist the receiver in understanding what they want/need (second center) so that they can communicate it (fifth center).

Cleansing Spin. Three minutes. Vetiver will release from the auric field anything that previously has not been spoken, or was said in a harsh or unhealthy way. It also completes the release of any thoughts and feelings processed during the session while sealing and protecting the auric field for negative influences.

Grounding Wave. Two minutes. Vetiver helps to strengthen grounding and assists in the integration of the intended changes.

Sweep and Comb. Two minutes. Mist your receiver with lavender or rose, and gently sweep and comb their auric field.

Close Toes. Two minutes. With lavender on your hands, touch each toe, beginning with the smallest and moving up to the big toes. Visualize the energy centers closing to the size that will be best for your receiver during the rest of their day.

A Session for Spiritual Rejuvenation

Open Toes. One to two minutes. Put lavender and/or chamomile on your hands to help your receiver relax and be receptive to the session.

Head Hold. Three minutes. Elemi brings the experience of deep peace and clarity, and opens the receiver to a connection with the Divine.

It balances all the energy centers. Imagine lavender light flowing into the entire body.

Forehead Spread. Three minutes. In order to support this spiritual rejuvenation at an appropriate pace—not too fast, not too slow—place rosewood on your hands. Imagine the seventh center slowly opening, like a great, golden flower.

Brain Balance. Five minutes. Cedarwood releases worry, and any other negative thoughts that could interfere with the rejuvenation of spirit as it integrates deeply into the body. Visualize the golden light used in the Forehead Spread moving down through the body, mingling with the lavender light already there.

Grounding Wave. Three minutes. Vetiver directs the light and energy of spirit all the way down into the body, especially into the feet, and insures that the spiritual rejuvenation does not result in the receiver becoming confused.

Energy Ball. Two minutes. Essential oil of orange helps the body increase its energy so that it can fully contain and integrate the spiritual vibration now developing.

Energy Center Balancing. Five minutes. This technique, done with vetiver, completes the spiritual energy's integration throughout the energy centers and subtle bodies. Vetiver also clears and cleanses any old thought patterns that might resist the infusion of spiritual energy.

Sweep and Comb. Two minutes. Turning onto their back again, mist your receiver with lavender or rose, and gently sweep and comb their auric field.

Close Toes. Two minutes. With lavender on your hands, touch each toe, beginning with the smallest and moving up to the big toes. Visualize the energy centers closing to the size that will be best for your receiver during the rest of their day.

Ending the Session

Tell your receiver that you are going to go wash your hands, and they may just lie comfortably until you come back. As you wash your hands, imagine that anything you might have energetically absorbed from the receiver is running down the drain with the soap and water.

Re-enter the room quietly, and assist your receiver in sitting up. Offer a glass of cool water to drink. This has a grounding effect and helps them orientate to their surroundings. Suggest they drink plenty of water to assist in the integration of the session that will continue over the next seventy-two hours. Before they get up, make sure they are well grounded. If still a bit woozy, have them take a sniff of a thyme/orange blend, and put a drop of vetiver on the bottom of their feet. Remember, it is your responsibility to be certain they are relaxed when they leave, but also grounded.

Take a few moments to ask how they are doing. They may want to tell you how they are feeling now, or about something they experienced during the session. Don't get into a lengthy discussion, as this can dissipate the energy. If they have questions or comments that can wait, talk to them in the following day or two.

After the receiver has left, take the time to adjust back to ordinary reality. Spray your clearing and cleansing spray again for yourself and the room. Turn off the diffuser, blow out the candles. Offer a prayer of gratitude for all the energetic gifts just given and received.

Recommended Reading

How Can I Help? Stories and Reflections on Service, Ram Dass (New York: Knopf Publishing, 1985).

Compassion in Action, Ram Dass (New York: Crown Publishing, 1995).

The Ethics of Caring, Kylea Taylor (New York: Hanford Mead Publishing, 1995).

Energy Medicine, Donna Eden (New York: Tarcher Putnam, 1998).

Hands of Life, Julie Motz (New York: Bantam Books, 1998).

Holistic Aromatherapy, Ann Berwick (St. Paul, Minnesota: Llewellyn Publications, 1994).

Afterword

"People won't remember what you've said and people won't remember what you've done but people will remember how you made them feel." —Author unknown

Helping people to feel better is the purpose of giving subtle energy treatments. You now have all the information you need to begin experiencing this transformative, healing art. We hope that your practice of this work will bring you the same possibilities for joy, healing, and spiritual growth that it has given to us. We wish you peace, wisdom, and the knowledge that as you give, you are receiving beyond all measure. Blessings to you.

Appendix I:

Subtle Energy to Help Common Imbalances

Each hand position used in subtle energy therapy has a variety of applications. Below you will find those that we have found to be effective for certain common imbalances, learned through study, experience, and conversations with other practitioners. Experiment, practice, and discover how these may be of help to you and your receivers.

PHYSICAL

Backache: Windshield Wipers
Congestion: Cleansing Spin
Disorientation (following physical trauma): Grounding Wave
Earache: Forehead Spread
Feet, poor circulation: Grounding Wave
Feet, aching: Grounding Wave, Simple Hold
Headaches: Brain Balance, Forehead Spread
Legs, poor circulation: Grounding Wave
Legs, aching: Grounding Wave, Simple Hold
Nausea: Grounding Wave
Travel sickness: Grounding Wave
Vision problems: Forehead Spread

PSYCHOLOGICAL

Anger: Grounding Wave
Confusion: Grounding Wave, Brain Balance, Forehead Spread
Creative Blocks: Brain Balance
Depression: Brain Balance
Disorientation (following mental or emotional trauma): Grounding Wave
Fear: Grounding Wave, Windshield Wipers
Grief: Simple Hold over the Heart center, Head Hold, Grounding Wave, Energy Center Balancing
Memory loss: Forehead Spread
Rigid thoughts: Forehead Spread

Spaciness: Grounding Wave, Brain Balance
Unreleased emotions: Cleansing Spin
Unreleased ideas and thoughts: Cleansing Spin
Obsessive thinking/worry: Brain Balance, Forehead Spread

ENERGETIC (SPIRITUAL)
Blocked (spiritual energy can't enter): Forehead Spread
Congested subtle bodies (all levels): Cleansing Spin
Disconnection (spirit from body): Grounding Wave
Disconnection (logical mind from spiritual perspective): Forehead Spread
Imbalance between intuitive and rational mind: Brain Balance
Insecure/feeling unsafe: Grounding Wave
Spiritual rigidity: Forehead Spread

Appendix II:
Quick Reference to Basic Hand Positions

1. *Open Toes/Close Toes*

   KEY PURPOSE To begin and end a subtle energy session by opening and closing the energy centers.

   PHYSICAL To link physical and subtle bodies together so subtle energy therapy can work on all levels.

   PSYCHOLOGICAL Balances.

   ENERGETIC/SPIRITUAL Balances.

2. *Head Hold*

   KEY PURPOSE To initiate deep relaxation, open receiver to healing energy, refresh all organs and energy centers, and clarify thoughts.

   PHYSICAL To ease vision problems, sore throats, tight jaws, headaches, and earaches.

   PSYCHOLOGICAL Relieves confusion, and obsessive and rigid thoughts. Useful for learning difficulties, memory loss, over-intellectualization, apathy, greed, nightmares, and shyness.

   ENERGETIC/SPIRITUAL Helps to connect the overly logical mind with a spiritual perspective. Allows spiritual and healing capabilities to enter.

3. *Forehead Spread*

   KEY PURPOSE To balance mental activities, and open receiver to healing energy.

   PHYSICAL Useful for headaches, vision problems, and sinus problems.

   PSYCHOLOGICAL Helps to clear confusion, worry, obsessive thoughts, doubt, mental conflict, creative blocks, problems in learning, and apathy.

   ENERGETIC/SPIRITUAL Helps to establish connection with spiritual path. Eases fear, confusion, or anger about religion and/or spirituality. Helps recognition of and response to intuition.

4. *Combing & Smoothing the Auric Field*

KEY PURPOSE To balance, clear, and seal the auric field, especially after a session. To promote a general sense of well-being by soothing and comforting the subtle bodies.

PHYSICAL Helps uncomfortable physical states such as sunburn, skin rashes, and irritation due to stress or worry.

PSYCHOLOGICAL Eases uncomfortable emotional states such as fear, anger, or grief.

ENERGETIC/SPIRITUAL Helps to repair an auric field damaged by physical or emotional trauma. Supports a healthy boundary during times of negative influences from relationships or toxic physical surroundings.

5. *Filling*

KEY PURPOSE To restore physical, mental, and emotional vibrancy and energy.

PHYSICAL Relieves exhaustion and fatigue.

PSYCHOLOGICAL Eases emotional and mental exhaustion, lack of joy, burn-out, stress, and emotional emptiness.

ENERGETIC/SPIRITUAL Gently increases the energy in the subtle bodies.

6. *Simple Hold*

KEY PURPOSE To bring an area into energetic balance so that the body's natural healing ability can unfold.

PHYSICAL Addresses all physical symptoms for which subtle energy is used.

PSYCHOLOGICAL Helps any symptom of mental or emotional imbalance such as worry, confusion, excessive thoughts, shock, moodiness, or exhausted nerves.

ENERGETIC/SPIRITUAL Helps to initiate and increase spiritual awareness.

7. *Brain Balance*

KEY PURPOSE To balance the intuitive and rational sides of the brain.

PHYSICAL Useful to relieves headaches and vision problems.

PSYCHOLOGICAL Relieves creativity blocks, obsessive thoughts or worry, depression, confusion, over-intellectualization, lack of imagination, and inability to visualize or remember dreams.

ENERGETIC/SPIRITUAL Helps to clear, open, and expand the mind.

8. *Energy Ball*

KEY PURPOSE To restore and strengthen physical, mental, and emotional energy.

PHYSICAL Relieves physical fatigue and exhaustion. Supports the immune system.

PSYCHOLOGICAL Eases emotional fatigue and exhaustion, low self-esteem, apathy, fear, despondency, hopelessness, indecision, and lack of joy.

ENERGETIC/SPIRITUAL Gently increases the energy in the subtle bodies.

9. *Windshield Wipers*

KEY PURPOSE To gently massage and balance the physical and subtle bodies.

PHYSICAL Eases lower back tension, as well as general physical tension. Stimulates lymph and blood circulation. Helps relieve constipation.

PSYCHOLOGICAL Soothes stress, anxiety, and mood swings.

ENERGETIC/SPIRITUAL Supports all energy centers, grounds, and helps to bring the spirit fully into the body.

10. *Grounding Wave*

KEY PURPOSE To connect, balance, and ground the body and mind.

PHYSICAL Helps to relieve headaches, dizziness, chilliness, panic attacks, and the trauma of physical shock.

PSYCHOLOGICAL Eases confusion, lack of concentration, disconnection from feelings, fear, hysteria, emotional or mental shock, worry, and general stress. Strengthens the left brain (rational mind).

ENERGETIC/SPIRITUAL Helps the spirit to reconnect with the body after meditation or deep spiritual work. Strengthens the first energy center, integrating the physical with the spiritual.

11. *Cleansing Spin*

KEY PURPOSE To clear all levels of the auric field after releasing physical and/or emotional distress.

PHYSICAL Does not apply to the physical body.

PSYCHOLOGICAL Releases negative emotions such as fear, anger, jealousy, or greed. Clarifies and focuses the mind.

ENERGETIC/SPIRITUAL Releases negative energy from all levels of the auric field.

12. *Energy Center Balancing*

KEY PURPOSE To promote an awareness of integrated wholeness, peace, and energy.

PHYSICAL To relieve any physical symptoms related to the energy centers such as: first—weight problems, second—menstrual problems, third—indigestion, fourth—circulation problems, fifth—hearing problems, sixth—impaired visions, and seventh—headaches.

PSYCHOLOGICAL To relieve any mental or emotional symptoms related to the energy centers such as: first—fear or apathy, second—poor boundaries, third—hyperactivity, fourth—jealousy, fifth—talking too much, sixth—poor memory, and seventh—confusion.

ENERGETIC/SPIRITUAL Relieves the congestion or constriction of energy centers. Promotes spiritual balance.

Appendix III:

Listening to the Oils

Chapter 3 discusses how the subtle properties of essential oils are determined, and includes an exercise called "Listening to the Oils." This fill-in form is for your convenience when practicing this exercise.

Holding the Oil:

Color: Texture:
Feeling: Sound:
Memory:
Fragrance: (May be different than the oil itself.)

Smelling the Oil:

Do you like or dislike the aroma?
Is there any place or places in your body that are affected by this fragrance?
Is there an energy center that is touched or stimulated?
Does it make you feel relaxed or energized?
Do you receive any sense impressions:
Color: Texture: Memory:
Shape: Image:
Temperature: Sound:

A "Conversation"

The responses may come in any sense—words, feelings, images, or sounds.
Complete this statement: "I am _____."
What are your subtle properties?
What energy center are you most connected with?
What are your energy gifts?
What are your spiritual gifts?
Is there anything about you that you want me to know?
Is there anything you want to communicate to me now?

Appendix IV:

Quick Reference to Key Essential Oils Used in Subtle Energy Therapy

The following oils are those listed in Chapter 3 as the Basic, Intermediate, and Advanced Oils used in subtle energy therapy. They are in alphabetical order, not in order of importance.

Angelica: Grounds. Connects us with angelic guidance.

Benzoin: Grounds and comforts. Steadies and focuses the mind for meditation or prayer.

Bergamot: Brings in positive energy. Promotes love. Eases grief.

Cedarwood: Clears and cleanses a room. Brings in positive energy. Grounds. Strengthens confidence.

Chamomile, German: Calms. Promotes the calm speaking of truth. Balances emotions.

Chamomile, Roman: Calms. Promotes patience. Eases grief and sadness.

Champaca: Energizes and balances the auric field and energy centers.

Clary Sage: Calms. Uplifts. Inspires. Helps us to see inwardly more clearly.

Coriander: Speeds the healing process. Promotes creativity and confidence.

Elemi: Grounds. Balances the worldly and spiritual life.

Eucalyptus: Clears and cleanses a room. Dissipates energy blockages. Balances emotions.

Frankincense: Grounds. Calms. Comforts. Promotes meditative states.

Geranium: Balances. Calms. Promotes harmony and happiness in relationships.

Grapefruit: Disperses emotional energy blockages. Promotes confidence. Increases intuition.

Immortelle: Disperses energy blockages. Promotes compassion. Activates right side of the brain.

Jasmine: Calms. Uplifts. Inspires. Promotes love, sensuality, creativity, and intuition.

Juniper: Clears and cleanses a room. Protects against negativity. Disperses energy blockages.

Lavender: Useful in all energy treatments to relax and balance. Brings in positive energy.

Lemon: Clears and cleanses a room. Promotes mental clarity. Clears emotional confusion.

Marjoram: Comforts. Promotes confidence. Helps us accept deep emotional loss.

Melissa: Promotes emotional clarity. Relieves emotional blocks due to grief.

Myrrh: Strengthens and supports. Grounds. Eases sorrow and grief. Supports spiritual journeys.

Neroli: Brings in positive energy. Eases grief. Promotes communication with the spiritual world.

Oakmoss: Grounds. Increases sense of prosperity and security.

Orange: Brings in positive energy. Promotes joy. Moves stagnated energy.

Palmarosa: Helps all levels of healing. Comforts the heart. Develops wisdom.

Patchouli: Grounds. Soothes. Strengthens. Relaxes. Opens the feet energy centers.

Peppermint: Promotes healthy self-esteem and clarity in communication. Inspires.

Rose: Promotes creativity, love, compassion, joy, and a sense of well-being. Inspires faith.

Rosemary: Clears and cleanses a room. Strengthens and centers. Protects from negative influences.

Rosewood: Brings in positive energy. Disperses energy blockages. Opens us to spirituality.

Sandalwood: Calms and comforts. Promotes healthy self-esteem. Quiets the mind. Promotes states of higher consciousness.

Spikenard: Promotes sense of hope. Comforts the heart. Increases spiritual love and devotion.

Thyme: Clears energy blockages. Relieves fear. Promotes self-confidence and courage.

Vetiver: Clears and cleanses a room. Grounds. Calms. Protects the auric field. Promotes wisdom.

Yarrow, blue: Provides protection. Promotes courage.

Appendix V:

Quick Reference to Subtle Energy Techniques and Key Essential Oils

The following are some of the ways essential oils are used during a subtle energy session. This is not an exhaustive list as there are many more applications and additional oils that could be used. The information here is to provide a quick reference for the most common applications and the oils associated with those applications.

To clear and cleanse the room or yourself:
> Use in a diffuser or as a spray.
> Cedarwood, eucalyptus, juniper, pine, lavender, dill, rosemary, lemon.

To promote positive energy:
> Use in a diffuser or as a spray.
> Bergamot, cedarwood, lavender, orange, neroli, petitgrain, rose, rosewood, vetiver.

Combinations of essential oils that both cleanse the room and bring in positive energy:
> Use in a diffuser or as a spray.
> Lavender/cedarwood/orange, lemon/orange, pine/rosewood.

To set up boundaries to provide protection:
> Use as anointing oils or spray.
> Fennel, rosemary, juniper, lemon, hyssop, vetiver.

To ask for guidance:
> Use as an anointing oil. Place one drop on the sixth energy center.
> Cedarwood, neroli, rose, jasmine, angelica, German chamomile, Roman chamomile, lavender, geranium, cistus, frankincense.

To link the hands to Heart energy:
>Use as an anointing oil.
>Rose and lavender together. Anoint your hands and heart before working on the receiver.

To activate your hands and make them more sensitive:
>Use as an anointing oil.
>Lavender.

To ground yourself before working on a receiver or to ground the receiver:
>Use as an anointing oil or spray. Apply to the feet energy centers.
>Patchouli, vetiver, oakmoss.

To help dissolve or release energy blockages:
>Use as a spray or an anointing oil.
>Juniper, black pepper, rosemary, silver fir, grapefruit, immortelle, eucalyptus.

192

To quiet the mind and promote a meditative state to better receive healing energy:
>Use in a diffuser, as a spray, or as an anointing oil.
>Sandalwood, frankincense, cedarwood.

To seal the auric field after energy healing work:
>Use as a spray or anointing oil.
>Rose.

To assist the Base energy center:
>Use as a spray or anointing oil.
>Benzoin, cedarwood, marjoram, myrrh, oakmoss, patchouli, sandalwood, vetiver.

To assist the Sacral energy center:
> Use as a spray or anointing oil.
> Cardamon, coriander, neroli, geranium, jasmine, orange, rose, ylang ylang.

To assist the Solar Plexus energy center:
> Use as a spray or anointing oil.
> Ginger, juniper, peppermint, rosemary, rosewood, tea tree, petitgrain.

To assist the Heart energy center:
> Use as a spray or anointing oil.
> Bergamot, immortelle, jasmine, lavender, marjoram, melissa, palmarosa, rose, spikenard.

To assist the Throat energy center:
> Use as a spray or anointing oil.
> German chamomile, Roman chamomile, fennel, geranium, myrrh, peppermint.

To assist the Third Eye energy center:
> Use as a spray or anointing oil.
> Basil, bay laurel, cedarwood, clary sage, fir, frankincense, immortelle, jasmine, juniper, lemon, palmarosa, peppermint, rosemary.

To assist the Crown energy center:
> Use as a spray or anointing oil.
> Angelica, cedarwood, elemi, frankincense, galbanum, lavender, neroli, myrrh, rose, rosemary, rosewood, sandalwood, spikenard.

Bibliography

A Gift For Healing, Deborah Cowens (New York: Crown Trade Paperbacks, 1996).

A Handbook for Light Workers, David Cousins (Dartmouth, England: Barton House, 1993).

Accepting Your Power to Heal: The Personal Practice of Therapeutic Touch, Dolores Kreiger, Ph.D. (Santa Fe, NM: Bear and Company Publications, 1993).

Affirmations, Cathy Guiswite (New York: Andrews and McMeel, 1996).

Anatomy of the Spirit, Carolyn Myss (New York: Harmony Books, 1996.)

Aromatherapy: A Complete Guide to the Healing Art, Kathy Keville and Mindy Green (Freedom, CA: The Crossing Press, 1995).

Aromatherapy for Vibrant Health and Beauty, Roberta Wilson (Garden City Park, NY: Avery Publishing Group, 1995).

Aromatherapy for Healing the Spirit, Gabriel Mojay (New York: Henry Holt and Company, 1996).

Aromatherapy: Scent and Psyche, Peter Damian and Kate Damian (Rochester, VT: Healing Arts Press, 1991).

Buffalo Woman Comes Singing, Brooke Medicine Eagle (New York: Ballantine Books, 1991).

Aromatherapy: A Lifetime Guide to Healing with Essential Oils, Valerie Gennari Cooksley (Englewood Cliffs, NJ: Prentice Hall, 1996).

Compassion in Action, Ram Dass (New York: Harper and Row, 1998).

Creative Visualization, Shakti Gawain (Berkeley, CA: Whatever Publishing, 1978).

Eastern Body, Western Mind, Anodea Judith (New York: Harper and Row, 1998).

Energy Medicine, Donna Eden (New York: Tarcher/Putnam, 1998).

Empowerment Through Reiki, Paula Horan (Twin Lakes, WI: Lotus Light Publications, 1990).

Full Catastrophe Living, Jon Kabat-Zinn, Ph.D. (New York: Dell Publishing, 1990).

Hands of Life, Julie Motz (New York: Bantam Books, 1998).

Hands-On Healing, Jack Angelo (Rochester, VT: Healing Arts Press, 1997).

Healers on Healing, Edited by Richard Carlson (New York: Tarcher Putnam, 1995).

Healing with Love, Leonard Laskow, M.D. (New York: Harper Collins, 1992).

Healing Words, Larry Dossey (New York: Harper-Collins, 1993).

How Can I Help? Stories and Reflections on Service, Ram Dass (New York: Knopf Publishing, 1985).

Hypnosis For Change, Josie Hadley and Carol Staudacher (Oakland, CA: New Harbinger Publishing, 1991).

Infinite Mind, Valerie V. Hunt (Malibu, CA: Malibu Publications, 1989).

Inner Knowing, Edited by Helen Palmer (New York: Tarcher Putnam, 1998).

Magical Aromatherapy, Scott Cunningham (St. Paul, MN: Llewellan Publishing, 1995).

Pendulum Power, Greg Neilsen and Joseph Polansky (New York: Harper Collins, 1987).

Psychic Protection, William Bloom (New York: Simon and Schuster, 1996).

Sacred Space: Clearing and Enhancing the Energy of Your Home, Denise Linn (New York: Ballantine Books, 1995).

Sevenfold Journey, Anodeath Judith and Selene Vega (Freedom, CA: Crossing Press, 1993).

Spiritual Cleaning, Draja Mickaharic (York Beach, ME: Samuel Weiser, Inc., 1982).

Subtle Aromatherapy, Patricia Davis (England: C. W. Daniel Company Limited, 1991).

Subtle Energy, William Collinge, Ph.D. (New York: Warner Books, 1998).

The Chakras and the Human Energy Field, S. Karcgulla and D. Kunz (Wheaton, IL: Theosophical Publishing House, 1976).

The Essence of Magic, Mary K. Greer (Van Nuys, CA: Newcastle Publishing, 1993).

The Ethics of Caring, Kylea Taylor (New York: Hanford Mead Publishing, 1995).

The Healing Energy of Your Hands, Michael Bradford (Freedom, CA: The Crossing Press, 1993).

The Healing Power of Aromatherapy, Hasnain Walji, Ph. D. (Rocklin, CA: Prima Publishing, 1996).

The Illustrated Encyclopedia of Essential Oils, Julia Lawless (Rockport, MA: Element Books, 1995).

The Inward Arc, Frances Vaughan (Nevada City, CA: Blue Dolphin Publishing, Inc., 1995).

The Light Inside the Dark, John Tarrant (New York: Harper Collins, 1998).

The Personal Aura, D. Kunz (Wheaton, IL: Theosophical Publishing House, 1991).

The Pendulum Kit, Sig Longren (New York: Fireside Books, 1990).

The World of Aromatherapy, Edited by Jeanne Rose and Susan Earle (Berkeley, CA: Frog, Ltd., 1996).

Vibrational Medicine, Dr. Richard Gerber (Santa Fe, NM: Bear and Company Publications, 1988).

Wheels of Light, Rosalyn Bruyere (New York: Fireside, 1994).

Wheels of Life, Anodea Judith (St. Paul, MN: Llewellyn Publications, 1996).

Your Hands Can Heal, Ric A. Weinman (New York: Penguin Books, 1992).

Your Healing Hands, Richard Gordon (Berkeley, CA: Wingbow Press, 1978).

Index

200

in subtle energy therapy, 80
subtle properties of, 62
undiluted, 34
for Windshield Wipers
technique, 99
Lemon
for affecting
consciousness, 111
as basic essential oil, 72
for clearing and
cleansing, 109
for energy boundaries, 110
quick reference, 188
subtle properties of, 62
Lemongrass, 33, 62
Lemon verbena, 33
Leptospermum, 62
Lime, 62
Limits, respecting, 162
Listening, active, 163–64
"Listening to the Oils"
exercise, 49–51, 185
Lovage, 63

M
Magnolia, 63
Mandarin, 63
Mangoginger, 63
Marjoram
as intermediate essential
oil, 73
quick reference, 188
subtle properties of, 63
Massage oils, 35
Mastic, 63
Maury, Margarite, 29
Meadowsweet, 63
Meerfenchel, 63
Melissa
as advanced essential oil, 73
chemical make-up of, 33

for Energy Ball
technique, 98
quick reference, 188
subtle properties of, 64
Mental body, 14, 15
Mental well-being, 139–40
Merton, Thomas, 146
Mimosa, 64
Misters, 35, 108, 112
Monarda, 64
Montague, Ashley, 5–6
Mugwort, 36
Music, 150
Myrrh
as intermediate essential
oil, 73
quick reference, 188
subtle properties of, 64
for Windshield Wipers
technique, 99
Myrtle, 64

N
Narcissus, 64
National Association of
Holistic Aromatherapy,
29, 41
Native Americans
ceremonies, 46
healers, 5
Neroli
as advanced essential oil, 73
in cosmetic applications, 28
for guidance, 111
for positive energy, 110
quick reference, 188
subtle properties of, 65
Neu, Dianne, 78
Niaouli, 65
Nigella seeds, 65
Nurse Healers-Professional
Association Cooperative, 20
Nutmeg, 65

O
Oakmoss
as advanced essential oil, 73
for Grounding Wave
technique, 100
quick reference, 188
subtle properties of, 65
for Windshield Wipers
technique, 99
Open Toes/Close Toes
technique, 86–88
aromatherapy for, 88
quick reference, 181
visualization and color
exercise for, 88
Opopanax, 65
Orange
as basic essential oil, 72
for Energy Ball
technique, 98
for Filling technique, 92
for positive energy, 110
quick reference, 188
subtle properties of, 65
for Windshield Wipers
technique, 99
Oxides, 33
P
Palmarosa
for Combing and
Smoothing the Auric
Field technique, 91–92
as intermediate essential
oil, 73
for Open Toes/Close Toes
technique, 88
quick reference, 188
subtle properties of, 66
Paraphrasing, 163
Pastinak, 66
Patchouli
for Grounding Wave
technique, 100
as intermediate essential
oil, 73

203

Biographies

Joni Keim Loughran has been working in the alternative health field since 1976 as a practitioner, educator, and author. She has certificates in massage, wholistic health sciences, aromatherapy, flower essence therapy, therapeutic touch, and energy healing. Joni has a private practice in Sonoma County, California, and is the co-founder of Light-Touched™, an energy healing system that employs the use of vibrational modalities.

Ruah Bull, m.a. has been working in the healing arts since 1978, and holds masters degrees in psychology and education. She is certified in aromatherapy, energy healing, and hypnotherapy. She is on the teaching faculty of the Transformational and Healing Arts Institute in Santa Rosa, California, and Twin Lakes College of the Healing Arts in Santa Cruz. Ruah is the co-founder of Light-Touched™, and has a private practice that specializes in assisting people with the emotional, mental, and physical initiations occurring during spiritual emergence.